Continuing Care
Retirement Communities

Continuing Care
Retirement Communities

Sylvia Sherwood
Hirsch S. Ruchlin
Clarence C. Sherwood
and Shirley A. Morris

The Johns Hopkins University Press ▪ Baltimore and London

The Johns Hopkins University Press
2715 North Charles Street
Baltimore, Maryland 21218-4319
The Johns Hopkins Press Ltd., London

Library of Congress Cataloging-in-Publication Data

Continuing care retirement communities/Sylvia Sherwood . . . [et al.].
    p.   cm.
  Includes bibliographical references and index.
  ISBN 0-8018-5434-2 (alk. paper)
    1. Life care communities — United States.   2. Aged — Long-term
care — United States.   I. Sherwood, Sylvia.
HV1454.2.U6C64   1997
362.1'6'0973 — dc20   96-22807

A catalog record for this book is available from the
British Library.

To the CCRC residents who participated in this study

Contents

Acknowledgments

We appreciate the funding support of the Health Care Financing Administration (HCFA) for the Evaluation of "Life Continuum of Care" Residential Centers in the United States (HCFA Cooperative Agreement CA 18-C-98672) and of the National Institute on Aging (NIA) for the High Risk Elders and Community Residence Study (NIA Grant RO1 AGO7820).

We also give thanks to the Research and Training Institute of the Hebrew Rehabilitation Center for Aged (HRCA) for encouragement and generous financial contributions to support the completion of this book.

We especially want to thank Dr. Judith Sangl, our project officer, for the Evaluation of "Life Continuum of Care" Residential Centers in the United States at HCFA, for her assistance and encouragement in this endeavor and Dr. John N. Morris, of the HRCA Research and Training Institute, particularly for his contributions to the economic analysis.

Many thanks to all the participating sites for their cooperation, especially the residents and staff who gave their valuable time and cooperation to this project, and to the research interviewers who gathered the data at these sites: Randy Halvorsen, Richard Oyler, Michael Vecellio, and Arlene Veliz. We want to acknowledge the efforts of Margaret Bryan, Ellen Gornstein, Monir Hossain, and Bernice MacLean, of the HRCA Research and Training Institute, and Daniel Nash, of the HRCA Information Systems Department. We also want to thank Herbert Weiss, Dr. David Levine, and Edie Mueller for editorial assistance with one or more chapters of this volume.

Continuing Care
Retirement Communities

ONE

Exploring the CCRC Phenomenon

As a result of advances in medicine, more Americans than ever before are surviving into old age. The segment of the population of age 85 and over is increasing at the fastest rate, followed by those aged 75 through 84 and 65 through 74 (Gunts 1994). Although many Americans age 65 and older remain in good health, the prevalence of functional and cognitive impairments increases sharply with age, especially for the older segments of the elderly population. In 1990, U.S. health care expenditures for nursing home care climbed to $53 billion, more than two and one-half times the amount spent in 1980; $6.9 billion was spent in 1990 on home health care, more than five times the amount spent in 1980 (Somers 1993).

Public awareness of the increased incidence of age-related chronic disease and degenerative conditions, as well as the escalating cost for those needing nursing home care, has brought the issue of long-term care costs into sharp focus. Older Americans also have cause for concern. Although Medicaid-eligible elderly persons might have access to government assistance for home health and nursing home costs, the financial burden for care falls on the shoulders of older people who are above the poverty line. When nursing home care is needed, elderly persons who are financially solvent find themselves forced to "spend down" their financial resources and savings until they reach the income level that qualifies them to become eligible for Medicaid (Cohen et al. 1987; Gornick et al. 1985).

At the same time, recognition of the potential benefits of housing features that can enhance functioning — such as site location, barrier-free design, enlightened management, and the integration of housing and supportive services — has led to the proliferation of planned housing options for older persons. Options range from senior housing projects and retirement communities that cater primarily to functionally independent elderly people to small board-and-care homes (often referred to as residential care or domiciliary care) for functionally and/or cognitively impaired older adults (Lawton 1988; Sherwood et al. 1988; Sherwood and Morris in press; Weeden et al. 1986).

A number of these housing options take into consideration potential changes in service needs which occur as an individual ages. For example, since the 1970s, congregate housing projects have developed, particularly in public and nonprofit-sponsored housing financed under Section 202 of the National Housing Act (Sherwood and Morris in press). However, when a tenant can no longer function at a satisfactory level with the types and quantity of services available, the individual must move out.

Continuing care retirement communities (CCRCs), sometimes called lifecare communities, represent another type of living arrangement which addresses specifically the problems associated with age-related disabilities. But this housing option goes further than congregate housing in responding to the needs of elderly persons as their health deteriorates and they need long-term care services. CCRCs can be described as planned communities that blend desirable housing, amenities, social activities, and health-related services (Cassel 1993; Sherwood et al. 1989; Somers 1993). CCRCs incorporate a continuum-of-care perspective, allowing residents to "age in place." The American Association of Homes for the Aging (AAHA), renamed the American Association of Homes and Services for the Aging (AAHSA) in 1994, has taken a major interest in developing information about CCRCs. From the early 1980s, this organization has been involved not only in data collection about CCRC facilities but also in such activities as developing directories, consumer guides, model regulations, and standards for voluntary accreditation of CCRCs. In 1988, the AAHA *National Continuing Care Directory* defined four essential characteristics of a CCRC (Raper and Kalicki 1988):

- a combination of residence, services, and nursing care as part of the long-term contract (a continuum of care);
- commitment to a community, as evidenced by a long-term contract, usually for the rest of the resident's life;
- residential care and nursing care in one location, coordinated or managed by the administrator;
- contracts that guarantee nursing care (through entrance and monthly fees), at a minimum, access to such care, and at a maximum, covering the full cost of nursing home care.

The contractual agreement between resident and management thus guarantees residents access to appropriate living arrangements within the same community as their health needs change. The entrance fee and monthly fees represent a form of prepayment for at least some of the services to be provided; essentially they are a type of insurance for the retirement years. The 1992 edition of *Continuing Care Retirement Communities: An Industry in Action* estimated that in 1990, there were between seven hundred and eight hundred entry-fee CCRCs, ranging from facilities that provide full coverage of nursing services to those supplying nursing care strictly on a fee-for-service basis (AAHA and Ernst and Young 1992).

It should be noted that although the entry fee might be substantial, the resident generally has no equity in the property. Rather, what has been purchased is a contractual agreement between the CCRC and resident (or a couple) in which the individual is provided with a specified type of apartment and ancillary services and a type of long-term care insurance guaranteeing, at a minimum, *access* to skilled nursing care when needed (usually in nursing home beds in the CCRC's health facility) and, at maximum, *full coverage* of nursing home care (Raper and Kalicki 1988).

Over the years, a growing amount of information has been compiled about CCRCs, largely from mail surveys sent to facility operators. Although the focus of data collection from such surveys is on the characteristics of CCRC facilities, some information regarding the demographics of CCRC residents has been obtained from operators or their designees filling out survey questionnaires. Some of the studies appearing in the literature since the early 1980s also provide information about CCRC residents. To a large extent, however, the descriptions and analyses presented are based on specific case histories or small samples involving only one or very few selected CCRCs (Barbaro and Noyes 1984; Elliott and Elliott 1985; Fillenbaum 1981; Hartwigsen 1984–85; Hunt et al. 1983; Morrison et al. 1986; Netting 1991; Rabins et al. 1992; Stacey-Konnert and Pynoos 1992; Stephens et al. 1986; Thompson and Swisher 1983). Several studies have examined predictors of movement from an independent living arrangement to a more dependent health care setting, for example, admission into the CCRC nursing home (Cohen et al. 1989; Falconer et al. 1992; Feinauer 1987; Newcomer and Preston 1994). On the whole, however, there has been relatively little longitudinal research in which data about the residents themselves and their CCRC experience have been gathered directly from large samples of individuals of multiple facilities.

This book presents findings from a multifaceted longitudinal study in which data were obtained directly from almost two thousand residents in nineteen CCRCs. A wealth of information is presented about these residents, their reasons for entrance, and their experience in the CCRC. A series of analyses compares residents in two different types of CCRC. Comparisons are also made with older persons in the general community.

The remainder of this chapter serves several purposes. It provides a brief overview of the evolving CCRC industry and the study being reported. Also, to provide information and insights concerning the segment of the elderly population which CCRCs serve, and as a context for the analyses in the chapters that follow, data are presented in which residents are compared with their age peers in the general community.

A Historical Overview of an Evolving Industry

The continuing care concept is not new. Its roots can be traced to the social programs of England, Germany, and Scandinavia. Among the precursors of the CCRC were the medieval guilds, which were the beginnings of the premodern attempts by self-reliant people, through prior contributions, to insure themselves against losses arising from death, sickness, injury, or old age. Mutual aid societies and the English friendly societies were also organized for such purposes (Winklevoss et al. 1984).

In the United States special types of housing with health care provisions have been developing for more than a hundred years. Many CCRCs are private-sector outgrowths of homes for the aged established by religious orders and groups to provide shelter and care for their aging clergy and older and disabled congregation members for the rest of their lives. Models of sponsorship and ownership are proliferating, and large hospital and nursing home chains, hotels, and other proprietary firms are entering the CCRC market (Cohen et al. 1988a; Pastalan 1989). However, as of the early 1990s, the vast majority of CCRCs were still nonprofit private-sector ventures (AAHA and Ernst and Young 1992).

The development of the concept of insurance against accident and sickness and against the loss of income in the retirement years may have helped pave the way for considering the CCRC a viable living arrangement. The availability of Social Security and Medicare may also have fueled the growth of the CCRC market in the United States. A major expansion of the industry began in the 1960s, with a large increase occurring in the 1980s (Cassel 1993). The 1988 National Continuing Care Data Base survey (a joint project of the AAHA and Ernst and Young) indicates that by 1988 CCRCs were located in thirty-five states (Somers 1993). By 1991, three states had fifty or more CCRCs—Pennsylvania was reported to have seventy-one, California fifty-two, and Florida fifty. Other states were reported to have none, specifically Alaska, Maine, Mississippi, Montana, Nevada, North Dakota, Rhode Island, Utah, Vermont, West Virginia, and Wyoming (Netting et al. 1992). In the late 1980s, the number of new CCRCs in the planning and development stage was estimated to be increasing by about 15 to 20 percent each year (Cohen et al. 1988a). Compared with an estimated 100,000 to 200,000 persons living in seven hundred CCRCs in the mid 1980s, some researchers predict that there will be 1,500 CCRCs with nearly 450,000 elderly residents by the beginning of the twenty-first century (Cohen 1988).

With increased interest and continued growth of the CCRC industry, some states have enacted legislation that, at least theoretically, regulates CCRCs. A primary focus has been to protect residents by lessening the likelihood of CCRC bankruptcy (Netting et al. 1990). Before 1970, only California had enacted such legislation, but since then many states have established regulatory oversight of these communities. As of 1991, thirty-five states had CCRC statutes. However, there is no consistency across states in how CCRCs are defined, which department or state agency is responsible for implementing regulations, or which regulations are implemented (Netting and Wilson 1994). Although CCRCs are most often regulated as insurance products, some states have assigned industry oversight to social or human services, health, commerce, securities, community affairs, and the state office on aging. Some states that have statutes requiring CCRC oversight have not designated state oversight units; in others, oversight requires coordination among multiple departments (Netting et al. 1990, 1992; Netting and Wilson 1994).

Despite the basic characteristics that CCRCs have in common, facilities vary as to sponsorship/ownership, whether a management company is retained to operate the CCRC, the specification and frequency of supportive services (e.g., transportation, meals, housecleaning, flat linens supplied and/or laundered), amenities (e.g., swimming pool, hiking and walking trails, convenience store, beauty salon, bank), payment mechanisms and refund policies, and other aspects of the contractual obligation between the CCRC and its residents.

The CCRC concept has been, and still is, evolving. A major change pertains to the assumption of the financial risk of increased costs. During the initial development of CCRCs, some required only an entry fee, and the community assumed the entire financial burden of providing appropriate accommodations and care to residents. However, this approach proved to be financially unsound, as evidenced by the bankruptcy of a number of early CCRCs (U.S. Senate 1983). Today, the entry-fee-only arrangement has just about disappeared. Monthly fees are now standard in the industry, although some CCRC contracts put an upper limit on the monthly fee or limit the amount of increases allowable over specified periods of time. The contractual commitment of the resident to some type of ongoing payment in addition to an entry fee holds great appeal to facility operators because it links revenue to the resident's longevity and provides a buffer against the effects of inflation. Some CCRCs, particularly those opened before 1963, require per diem payments for nursing care (AAHA and Ernst and Whinney 1987). In some cases, the resident-facility contract stipulates a designated (and finite) time period for the contract rather than lifecare. Taking the concept of per diem payments to the extreme, some CCRCs offer nursing care on a market fee-for-service basis only.

In the Wharton School Survey conducted in the early 1980s, in which, for the first time, an attempt was made to identify and conduct an actuarial survey of CCRCs nationwide, communities operating totally on a fee-for-service arrangement for nursing care were not considered in the CCRC domain (Winklevoss et al. 1984). This was the case even if other aspects of care were in place, including a continuum of housing options and services within the community, with entry and monthly fees and guaranteed access to nursing home care. Reflecting the growth of the CCRC industry, however, the AAHA expanded its definition to include communities that offer nursing home care on a fee-for-service basis as long as *access* to long-term health services is guaranteed. A three-category classification of CCRC contracts was put forth based on the extent to which the entry and monthly fees provide for nursing home care without additional charges to residents (AAHA and Ernst and Whinney 1987; AAHA and Ernst and Young 1992):

- *All-inclusive or extensive contracts.* The contract is sometimes referred to as a *lifecare agreement.* This approach provides unlimited nursing home care as needed in return for the entry and monthly fees.
- *Modified contracts.* The contractual agreement provides a specified amount of nursing home care in return for the entry and monthly fees, for example, a specified number of days per year, but care beyond the agreed-upon time frame is charged either at a discounted rate or full fee-for-service rate.
- *Fee-for-service contracts.* The contract offers nursing home care at a full fee-for-service rate.

Theoretically, under contracts that include per diem payments for nursing care, facility owners minimize, and might even eliminate, their risk for care beyond the levels implicit in the entry and monthly fees. However, there is little indication from the literature or from anecdotal reports that residents, whether their CCRC offers fee-for-service, modified, or extensive contracts, have been actually asked to leave a CCRC because of their inability to pay the fees, especially when it is no fault of their own. A sizable number of the CCRC nursing homes are Medicaid certified, about half of the facilities listed in the 1988 AAHA *National Continuing Care Directory* (Raper and Kalicki 1988). These facilities have the Medicaid program available to provide funds after residents' assets and income become exhausted. Some CCRCs accumulate contributed funds to subsidize residents in the health center when necessary.

Although there had been a trend to move away from or reduce pooled risk as the major mechanism for financing nursing care during the 1970s and into the 1980s, interest in the all-inclusive CCRC seems to be increasing (Tell and Cohen 1990). The proportion of all-inclusive facilities among the CCRCs known to be in operation is increasing while the proportion of fee-for-service CCRCs is decreasing. In a 1991 survey (AAHA and Ernst and Young 1992), 43 percent of the responding CCRCs in 1990 were of the extensive (all-inclusive) type. About 28 percent were fee-for-service facilities only. Of those CCRCs opened between 1986 and 1991, 63 percent were extensive, and only 16 percent were fee-for-service. The trend toward all-inclusive CCRCs might in part be a reflection of market research findings indicating that, even in the face of it being more expensive, individuals are more likely to say they would choose a retirement community that protects them against long-term costs rather than one that does not (Tell and Cohen 1990).

The growth of the long-term care insurance market has also stimulated increased interest in the extensive CCRC. Links with insurance companies have been made, using this risk-pooling method as a way of minimizing some of the financial uncertainty about future costs for nursing home care. A number of CCRCs have negotiated with insurance companies to offer long-term care insurance packages to residents residing in the independent living units (ILUs). They are required to contract with the designated company to purchase long-term care insurance.

Another refinement in financing CCRC care, and an attractive feature for potential residents regardless of the type of CCRC, is the introduction of entry-fee refund policies. In the past, it has usually been the policy of facilities to provide for a probationary period within the first three years, after which no or very limited refunds would be available. Many CCRCs now offer refunds whenever the resident leaves, including a refund to the heirs upon the death of the resident. One estimate is that most newly written contracts provide a refund of 90 percent of the entry fee (Higgens 1992). However, to accommodate such a policy, fees (entry and/or monthly) are likely to be higher.

A small number of CCRCs recently opened or in the planning stage have embraced the concept of equity by marketing the facility as a type of a condominium or cooperative. Equity CCRCs can be all-inclusive, modified, or fee-for-service type facilities. As with entry-fee CCRCs, persons buying into the community must meet the CCRC financial and health eligibility requirements. In addition to owning the unit in a condominium or purchasing a share in a cooperative, residents pay a monthly fee to cover the costs of maintenance, recreation, amenities, and supportive services such as meals and housekeeping. The resident or heirs upon the death of the resident cannot sell the empty unit, but almost all or a set portion of the resale value—the money paid by the new owner who occupies the empty unit—is returned to the former resident or heirs. It is reported that in many of these CCRCs, the CCRC and resident share the appreciation on a resold unit (Magan 1993).

According to the American Association of Retired Persons (AARP) *Housing Report*, published in spring 1993, the National Continuing Care Data Base indicates that while others were in the development stage, only about a dozen equity CCRCs were in operation. At least a third of these facilities were in California, with more under development. The AARP report pointed to the potential growth of this model, noting that major retirement-housing developers, including the American Retirement Corporation, the Marriott Corporation, and Life Care Services, had plans for and/or already had communities under construction (Magan 1993).

Seeing the growing number of elderly persons who might at some point require long-term care services, for-profit developers are building rental communities that do not require an entry fee but have features that are similar to CCRCs. They offer, on a short-term lease basis, apartments with amenities such as recreational opportunities and coffee shop and a limited amount of supportive services, including one or more meals per day and weekly light housekeeping services, as part of a monthly fee. Residents, should they desire, also have an opportunity to purchase an increase in the frequency of these services as well as personal care and other health services. A continuum of housing options and services is usually on the same campus or nearby so that a resident needing a specific level of services could choose to move (for an increased fee) to a more supportive environment (i.e., a personal care home or nursing home in the same campus area, if beds become available).

However, these rental facilities do not necessarily have the same commitment to the aging-in-place concept, and residents cannot count on the protective features usually found in entry-fee CCRCs. The on-site health facilities are open to the public with no necessary provision to reserve beds for their tenants when needed. Apartment dwellers whose health deteriorates to the extent that they can no longer care for themselves adequately, even with the supportive services available, might be asked to move whether or not a bed is available in the health facility (although priority on the waiting list might be given to these tenants).

Rental facilities also do not generally appear to have any of the elements of pooled risk usually found in entry-fee CCRCs. Although these facilities deal with the supportive-service needs of their residents, they appear to have no commitment to keep residents or to serve their needs beyond the residents' ability to pay. Those who cannot afford this living arrangement are expected to leave. Similarly, there is little evidence of obligation to the community by the residents themselves (i.e., there is usually no community fund supported by the residents to ensure that persons who can no longer afford to live there will be able to remain).

Until the 1990s, communities that did not meet the four conditions specified by the AAHA were not considered CCRCs. By 1991, in recognition of the growth of this phenomenon, rental communities were being included in the National Continuing Care Data Base and referred to in a number of reports as a type of CCRC (AAHA and Ernst and Young 1992; Cassel 1993). As of 1992, analyses of CCRC industry trends using data from the National Continuing Care Data Base have involved entry-fee CCRCs only — facilities that have all four of the necessary CCRC characteristics specified in the AAHA 1988 directory. A 1992 report profiling industry trends asserted that analyses in subsequent editions will also include data on rental and equity arrangements (AAHA and Ernst and Young 1992). Including entry-fee, equity, and rental communities offering a continuum of care (including multilevel accommodations), the AAHA estimated that one thousand CCRCs were in operation at the end of 1991 (Somers 1993).

Rental communities that offer a continuum of services on a more traditional buyer-seller fee-for-service and first-come/first-served basis might be of interest to potential consumers, an ample reason for inclusion of rentals in the National Continuing Care Data Base. However, it is hoped that future reports profiling the CCRC industry will present data separately for entry-fee CCRCs. This will be important in helping researchers, CCRC developers, and operators to understand better the characteristics of planned communities that have a relatively stable population of residents. Such data will also allow comparisons to be made between entry-fee CCRCs and communities that offer a continuum of services which, at least conceptually, are less likely to have case management as part of the monthly services and are apt to have a more transitory population of elderly people.

In the study being reported in this book, we have included only those communities that have at least some level of pooled risk (reflected in the entrance and monthly fees), specifically facilities that offer long-term contracts, have a long-term commitment to their residents, and guarantee access to nursing home care when needed. We have excluded facilities that were established purely on a rental basis and in which pooled risk of any sort is absent.

In preparing for the "graying" of America, which will arguably be the major social dilemma of the first part of the twenty-first century, planners and policy makers will have to address the service needs and quality of life of the elderly population. New policy initiatives will need to address such issues as:

- ensuring access (direct and financial) both to long-term supportive community services and nursing home services when necessary;
- ensuring access (direct and financial) both to community-based social supports and adequate housing;
- without eliminating the benefits of an informal care network, ensuring access while addressing the elder person's need to retain locus of control (Estes 1993);
- integrating acute and long-term health care services; and
- addressing society's concern with the high costs of medical care and consequently the development of cost-conscious interventions (some would say, especially with regard to the perceived "high cost of dying").

CCRCs are attempting to address these issues, at least from the point of view of the elderly consumer. Information about the CCRC living arrangement in relation to its residents is of interest not only to the general field of gerontology, but also to policy makers and social planners, to groups wanting to develop a CCRC (particularly with respect to decisions regarding target populations and their characteristics), and to elderly persons themselves who are planning for their future and might be potential consumers of this type of living arrangement.

This CCRC Study

In the mid 1980s, a multifaceted longitudinal study was undertaken which involved approximately two thousand residents in nineteen CCRCs: four in Arizona and five each from the three states with the largest number of CCRCs — California, Florida, and Pennsylvania. In selecting CCRCs and their residents for study participation, an attempt was made to recruit an equal number of communities in which pooled risk (for nursing home care) was extensive (extended CCRCs) and those with more limited pooled risk (limited CCRCs). Of the nineteen participating CCRCs, nine were classified as extended CCRCs (those with *all-inclusive* or *extensive* contracts as defined by the National Continuing Care Data Base surveys); that is, they provided nursing home care on a virtually *unlimited* basis at no or little extra cost to the resident (e.g., additional charges for meal services were not ordinarily included in the monthly fee). The ten CCRCs providing less financial protection against high costs of long-term care were classified as limited CCRCs. They provided nursing home care on a full fee-for-service basis or on a discounted fee-for-service basis (e.g., compared with persons who were not CCRC residents but were admitted to the nursing facility), or they provided a limited period of nursing home coverage without additional charges before implementing services on a full or discounted fee-for-service basis (CCRCs with *modified* or *fee-for-service* contracts).[1]

This study gathered information about the organizational characteristics, operating costs, and contracts offered by the nineteen facilities. However, the bulk of data collection and analyses — and the focus of this book — pertains to residents of CCRCs. Most of the data regarding residents were gathered directly from interviews at two points of time (baseline and follow-up). The baseline (initial) interviews were begun in August 1986 and continued throughout the next year. The residents interviewed at the initial contact were contract holders in independent units (usually apartments, but in some CCRCs, cottages and town houses as well). Follow-up interviews were held about sixteen months later, with the last interviews completed by June 1989.

CCRC Resident Sampling Procedures, Data Collection, and Analysis

Sampling was conducted separately for residents of a year or more (longer-stay residents) and those in the CCRC for less than a year (recent residents). For the longer-stay sample, a random sample of eighty longer-stay apartment-dwelling residents at baseline was selected in each facility. The sample of recent residents included two subsamples. One consisted of up to the first twenty persons moving to the CCRC in the year of baseline data collection, which usually represented all such persons. These residents were contacted within approximately the first two weeks after they moved into the community. The second subsample consisted of a random sample of twenty residents from each of these participating facilities who had lived there more than two weeks but less than a year before the baseline interview. Most of the resident analyses involved elderly persons with baseline interviews.

This was not the case, however, for analyses pertaining to service

1. An additional facility originally considered to be a fee-for-service CCRC was dropped when it became apparent that it was a "rental" facility, with no assumption of pooled risk at any level.

utilization during the last year of life. Only a small number of sample members with baseline interviews had died between baseline and follow-up (a little more than 6 percent). Therefore, to help enlarge the sample for these analyses, CCRC residents who were not part of the representative CCRC samples but who died during 1985 were added to the last-year-of-life sample.

Data about residents were gathered from the in-depth baseline and follow-up interviews held with these sample members. Information gathered covered many areas, including demographic data, health and functional status, use of amenities, activities, social interaction and other personal characteristics, reasons for entrance, satisfaction with the CCRC experience, informal supports, and self-reported service utilization. For residents who had died (whether or not in the representative samples) and the few recent and longer-stay residents with baseline interviews who were alive but unable to respond at follow-up, special "proxy" follow-up interviews were held with family members, friends, or, in some cases, knowledgeable CCRC staff.

To the extent available, utilization and expenditure data were also obtained from the Health Care Financing Administration (HCFA) Medicare Automated Data Retrieval System (MADRS) Part A-Part B skeleton file. Information derived from this file was the data of choice for analyses pertaining to services, which was supplemented when necessary by self-reports on service utilization obtained from interviews with residents or their proxies. Because of the difficulty in obtaining MADRS data for a sufficient number of CCRC sample members who had died (and a comparison group from a sample of elderly persons residing in a traditional community, described below), a profile of hospital and nursing home utilization during the last year of life and the imputed cost was developed from data reported by family, friends, and/or knowledgeable staff.

Major analyses in this book pertain only to CCRC residents. Data from secondary sources also made cross-sectional and longitudinal comparisons possible between the CCRC samples and traditional-community residents regarding selected personal characteristics, quality-of-life outcomes, service utilization, and Medicare costs.

It should be noted that an age criterion was invoked for analyses comparing CCRC residents with traditional-community residents. It is clear from the National Continuing Care Data Base periodic surveys that CCRCs attract the older segments of the elderly population. In sharp contrast with the age distribution within the national population of persons 65 years of age and older, more than half of whom were under 70 in the mid 1980s (U.S. DHHS 1987; U.S. DHHS SSA 1985), the overwhelming majority of CCRC residents were at least 70 years of age (almost 90 percent were at least 75 years of age), with the residents well into their 70s (AAHA and Ernst and Whinney 1987; AAHA and Ernst and Young 1992; Winklevoss et al. 1984). In fact, of the CCRC sample members in this study, very few were under 70 years of age: of a baseline sample of 595 recent residents living in ILUs, only 38 were under 70 years of age; of 1,432 longer-stay residents, only 19 were under 70 years of age. Therefore, comparisons with traditional-community elderly persons in this study were restricted to those who were 70 years of age or older.

Comparison Samples/Data Sources

Although little exists in the literature to enable age-stratified comparisons between CCRC residents and elderly persons in the community, it was possible to use U.S. census data to analyze demographic characteristics. Although most census reports do not differentiate subgroups of the age category 65 and older, census data regarding the U.S. population 75 and older in 1980 were abstracted (Longino 1986). Using these data, descriptive cross-sectional comparisons were made between characteristics of persons 75 years of age and older in the national population and those of similar age in the CCRC samples. Comparisons with the national population in this age group were expanded further using 1984 economic data for elderly persons, and the data were broken down by age group subcategories, as reported by the Social Security Administration (U.S. DHHS SSA 1985).

More detailed cross-sectional and longitudinal comparisons in this study were possible using data collected as part of a longitudinal study initiated in 1982 by the Department of Social Gerontological Research at the Hebrew Rehabilitation Center for Aged in Boston (HRCA).[2] The study encompassed a representative sample of elderly persons in Massachusetts and enabled comparisons with older individuals living in the community. Comparable data in a variety of domains were available from two follow-up waves[3] of interviews (e.g., demographic, health and functional status, social interaction, informal supports, and self-reported service utilization). These Massachusetts study interviews were conducted eighteen months apart in overlapping time periods during which data were gathered from the CCRC samples. Furthermore, proxy data (usually from a spouse or child) regarding service utilization during

2. Supported in part by National Institute on Aging-supported HRCA-Harvard Teaching Nursing Home Grant AGO4390 and High Risk Elders and Community Residence Grant AGO7820.
3. The third and fourth waves of data collection in the study of elderly Massachusetts residents.

the last year of life were also available in this study for Massachusetts sample members who had died in the preceding year as well as for sample members who died between these two waves of interviews. This enabled an enlargement of a last-year-of-life sample comparable to sample selection in the CCRC study.

Supplementing the interview data collected in the Massachusetts study, efforts were made in the CCRC study to obtain information from the HCFA MADRS file for these samples. Interview and supplemental MADRS data regarding people in the Massachusetts sample who were 70 years or older and living in the community at the first of these two waves (approximating initial, or baseline, data collection in our study of CCRC residents) or who were in the last-year-of-life sample were used for comparisons between CCRC samples and a traditional population of elderly persons in this age group.

In analyses pertaining exclusively to the CCRC samples as well as in comparisons between the CCRC and older individuals living in the community, descriptive as well inferential statistical techniques were employed, including uncontrolled bivariate and more complex multivariate techniques. In analyses employing inferential statistics, differences at the p 0.05 level were considered significant. The specific statistical techniques employed differed depending upon the particular questions being addressed and, in each case, are specified as relevant to the presentation of study findings.

Except for cross-sectional analyses of baseline characteristics and service utilization, the samples consisted of elderly people who were alive and in the community at baseline and at follow-up. The particular sample or samples used, data sources, and the specific variables studied differed depending upon the particular analyses and are described as relevant in this chapter and in the chapters that follow.

The CCRC Population in Context

A picture of the baseline characteristics of the samples of recent residents (those in the CCRC community for less than a year) and longer-stay residents in apartments as well as comparisons of these samples with elderly people living in the community can provide insights as to the special nature of CCRC residents as well as a context for the analyses in the chapters that follow. Using data from the baseline interviews and secondary sources to enable comparisons with elderly persons in the community, the remainder of this chapter is devoted to filling out this picture.

Selected findings regarding demographic characteristics of the overall samples of CCRC apartment dwellers interviewed at baseline have been reported previously (Sherwood et al. 1989). These and other key features regarding the recent and longer-stay residents considered as a whole are summarized here. A series of cross-sectional comparisons of older age groups then follows.

Data Sources for Cross-sectional Comparisons

Comparable data from the following sources (mentioned previously) were analyzed:

1. Baseline interview data gathered in 1986 and early 1987 from random samples of CCRC residents in ILUs (apartments) in the nineteen study CCRCs, focusing in particular on comparisons involving recent residents ($N = 557$) and longer-stay residents ($N = 1,413$) who were 70 years of age and older at the initial interview (baseline), stratified into four separate age groups (70 through 74 years, 75 through 79 years, 80 through 84 years, and 85 years and older).
2. Selected secondary data pertaining to the Massachusetts study sample members who were 70 years or older, living in the community, and interviewed at an overlapping period with baseline interviews in the CCRC study ($N = 1,447$), stratified by the above four separate age groups.
3. Special abstractions of 1980 national census data regarding demographic characteristics of people 75 years and older and of 1984 economic data.

Types of Comparisons

To place CCRC residents in the national scene, data regarding the subsamples of 448 recent and 1,325 longer-stay residents who were 75 years of age and older at baseline were compared descriptively with respect to demographic characteristics abstracted from the 1980 national census data (detailed in Table 1.2 in a later section of this chapter). For analyses pertaining to economic status, data from the CCRC samples regarding three economic status variables were also compared with 1984 national data reported by the SSA for elderly community residents in this age group (one of which was a variable for which 1980 census data were presented as well). However, because of limited economic data collected at baseline for CCRC samples, data collected at follow-up interviews were used for the economic status comparisons. Estimates regarding incomes below and above the poverty level for the CCRC samples were based on SSA poverty-level criteria for the time period when these data were collected (see Appendix A for the algorithm used in making these estimates).

Involving a much broader range of variables, a more robust picture of CCRC residents compared with their age peers in the general community can be seen from separate age subgroup comparisons of characteristics of CCRC and Massachusetts sample members, including subgroups of sample members 70 through 74, 75 through 79, 80 through 84, and 85 and older years of age at baseline. Classifying variables into three broad categories, cross-sectional age-stratified comparisons were conducted for eighteen selected demographic characteristics; fifteen variables representing health conditions and key areas of functional status; and responses to seven miscellaneous questions regarding activities, social interaction, and areas of decision making and informal support. The specific variables will be described in the final sections of this chapter in which the data and key findings from age-stratification comparisons are presented (Tables 1.3, 1.4, and 1.5). For comparison purposes, the age-stratified comparisons of recent and longer-stay CCRC residents focus on the same age groups and involve the same sets of variables — demographic, health and functional status, and other life-style characteristics — as in comparisons across the Massachusetts and CCRC samples.

Age-Stratified Comparisons: Sample Sizes and Statistical Analyses

Illustrative of the sharp differences in age distributions between CCRC and traditional-community populations, except for persons 85 years of age and older among recent CCRC residents, the numbers in these representative samples increased steadily with age in the CCRC sample. In contrast, the numbers decreased steadily in the representative samples of elderly Massachusetts community residents. The sample sizes for comparisons in each of the age brackets starting with the group 70 through 74 years of age were as shown in Table 1.1.

Even when limited to persons 70 years of age and older, CCRC residents tended to be concentrated in the older age groups, whereas the elderly community residents in Massachusetts were concentrated in the younger age groups. The majority (65 percent) of the representative Massachusetts sample of community residents 70 years of age and older was between 70 and 79 years of age, whereas recent CCRC residents were concentrated in the groups between 75 and 84 years of age (62.5 percent), and longer-term CCRC residents were heavily concentrated in the oldest age groups, with close to three quarters (73.6 percent) 80 years of age or older at baseline.

In age-stratified comparisons of recent, longer-stay CCRC residents, and the Massachusetts community populations, chi-square (for analyzing differences in percentages) and analysis of variance techniques (for

Table 1.1 Sample sizes in age brackets

Age group (years)	CCRC resident sample sizes		Sizes of representative MA community samples
	Recent	Longer-stay	
70 to 74	109	88	496
75 to 79	165	285	444
80 to 84	183	465	311
85 and older	100	575	196

analyzing mean differences) were employed. Comparisons pertaining exclusively to recent and longer-stay CCRC residents utilized chi-square and t-test statistics, as appropriate.

Demographic Characteristics of the Overall CCRC Study Group

As has been found by others (AAHA and Ernst and Whinney 1987; Marans et al. 1984), data from the CCRC study sample members (regardless of age or date of entrance) clearly indicate that CCRCs tend to serve white, well-educated middle- to upper-middle-class people from the older segments of the elderly population (Sherwood et al. 1989, 1993). More than 98 percent in the sample were white. Almost half (48 percent) of recent residents and an even significantly larger proportion of longer-standing residents (53 percent) had graduated from college. Although recent entrants were likely to have higher incomes than those in the CCRC for a year or more, sizable proportions of both groups—as many as 52 percent of recent CCRC residents and 44 percent of those in the CCRC for a year or longer—had annual incomes of more than $30,000. As many as 75 percent of the recent and significantly more, 92 percent, of the CCRC apartment dwellers of a year or more were in the 75 and older age bracket at baseline.

The majority of CCRC apartment dwellers (68 percent of the recent and 78 percent of the longer-stay residents) were women—not an unusual finding for the older segment of the elderly population. Only about a third of the CCRC residents who had lived at the facility for a year or more (longer-stay residents), but more than half (55 percent) of the recent residents, were not living alone. (It is presumed that most of these persons were married at the time.) In fact, although seemingly more so than currently, a significantly smaller proportion of longer-stay (48 percent) residents were living alone even when they first joined the CCRC.

A significantly higher proportion of the longer-stay residents (13 percent) than the more recent residents (7 percent) had never been married. The mean age when joining the CCRC for longer-stay residents was actually younger than for recent residents (76.7 and 78.1 years of age, respectively). This age discrepancy is apparently accounted for by the larger proportion of longer-stay residents who had never been married since, in general, the average age at entrance of persons who had never married was younger — 74.4 years — than the 77.5 years at entrance of other residents.

Even though the majority of residents were women who were 75 years of age or older, most residents (85 percent) had worked outside the home during most of their adult life (with the same proportions found for recent and longer-stay residents). Of those who had worked for most of their adult lives, a large majority of CCRC residents (between 92 and 94 percent) appear to have been white-collar workers — to a large extent professionals (59 percent of those in the CCRC community for a year or more and 51 percent of the more recent residents), but there were also proprietors or managers and sales or clerical workers.

Although significantly more so for the longer-stay residents, the majority had no children living within a one-hour drive — 66 percent of recent residents and 74 percent of the longer-stay residents. In fact, a sizable proportion of the CCRC study samples did not have living children — more than a third (34 percent) of those in the recent and an even significantly larger proportion (42 percent) of the longer-stay residents.

Characteristics of Older CCRC Residents with National Data

Clearly, the characteristics of the CCRC sample members described above indicate that, in many respects, the CCRC residents were not representative of their age group in the general population. This conclusion is supported by comparisons of study data with national data regarding demographic characteristics of the elderly population 75 and over in the community at large. Descriptive comparisons were made regarding the following (unless otherwise specified, presented in terms of the percent with each characteristic): female; lives alone (by self); three marital status variables (married, widowed, and never married); four racial identification variables (white, black, Indian and Asian, and Hispanic); three educational status variables (high school graduate/higher level of education, one or more years of college, and mean number of years of schooling); three sources of income variables (employed full/ part time, income from Social Security, income from investments); and four economic status variables (income under $20,000, household income below the poverty-level threshold, household income at least twice the poverty level, and (rather than percentages) categorized median household income (see Table 1.2).

In some instances the recent residents but not the longer-stay CCRC residents and in others the longer-stay but not the recent residents were similar to the national population. Specifically, although the sex distribution of recent residents was somewhat similar to the national population for this age group, the proportion of females among the longer-term residents (78 percent) was much larger than the national population of 75 years of age or older (64 percent). Only a small minority in all groups had never been married, but twice the proportion of longer-stay CCRC residents in this age group (almost 13 percent) than their age counterparts in the national population (almost 7 percent), and more than three times as many as recent CCRC residents (4 percent), had never been married.

On the other hand, longer-stay residents as a whole looked more like the 75 and older age group in the national population than did the more recent residents in the percents widowed and married. More than half in the national and in the longer-stay CCRC populations were widowed (53 percent in each group), and only a minority (37 and 32 percent, respectively) were still married. Fewer than half (43 percent) of the CCRC residents of less than one year were widowed, and as many as 50 percent were married.

A larger proportion of both the recent and longer-stay CCRC residents who were 75 years of age or older lived alone (49 and 67 percent, respectively) than persons in this age group nationally (of which only about a third lived alone). It appears that the CCRC is taking the place of the informal network in giving residence and support services to elderly persons who become widowed and frail.

A number of differences exist between the national population 75 years of age and older and their age counterparts in the CCRC samples, regardless of the length of stay. Specifically, a lower proportion of CCRC residents, both recent (less than 2 percent) and longer-stay (1 percent), was nonwhite than that found in the national population of persons 75 years of age and older (almost 10 percent). The same pattern applies to persons of Hispanic origin (less than 1 percent of the CCRC but more than 2 percent of the national population).

The CCRC residents were a much better educated group than their counterparts in the general population. The national mean (average) educational level for this age group was less than high school, whereas the mean educational level of the CCRC residents was more than two years of college. Compared with only a minority in the general popula-

Table 1.2 Demographic characteristics of persons age 75 and older, by U.S. population and recent and longer-stay CCRC residents

Demographic characteristic	U.S. population 75+ (1980 N = 10,128,019)	CCRC population 75+	
		Recent (N = 448)	Longer-stay (N = 1,325)
Female (%)	64.4	67.6	78.0
Marital status			
Married (%)	37.0	50.0	32.1
Widowed (%)	53.4	43.1	53.4
Never married (%)	6.7	4.0	12.7
Live alone (%)	33.5	49.3	67.3
Race/ethnicity			
White (%)	90.8	98.4	99.0
Black (%)	7.4	1.1	0.7
Indian (%)	0.3	0.2	0.3
Asian (%)	0.8	0.2	0.0
Hispanic (%)	2.4	0.7	0.4

Educational status			
Mean years of schooling	14.7	14.4	9.2
High school graduate or more (%)	89.0	87.0	30.8
1+ years of college (%)	73.6	70.0	14.2
Employed (full or part time) (%)	2.4	2.5	5.0
Income sources			
Social Security (%)	95.2	96.4	80.5
Investments (interest, dividends, rent) (%)	94.5	96.6	39.3
Economic status			
Incomes under $20,000 (%)	24.4	18.1	72.1 (1984)
Categorized median household Income [1 = under $20,000; 2 = $20–29,999; 3 = $30–39,999; 4 = $40–49,999; 5 = $50,000+]	2.0	3.0	1.0 (1984)
Household income below poverty level threshold (%)	0.01	0.0	17.7 (1984) 16.5 (1980)
Household income at least twice the poverty level (1980) (%)	96.0	98.0	41.5 (1980)

Note. Except for 1984 income information, U.S. population data were excerpted from 1980 Census data reported in Longino (1986). 1984 income data were derived from Tables 10 and 51 in SSA Publication 13-11871, December 1985.

tion graduating from high school (31 percent) and an even smaller minority with one or more years of college (14 percent), a large majority of CCRC residents graduated high school (more than 85 percent), and more than 70 percent had at least some college.

Whereas very small proportions of the national (5 percent) and the CCRC populations (less than 3 percent) of this age group were still employed, sources of income and economic status differed dramatically. For example, the vast majority of the 75 years and older recent and longer-stay residents (approximately 95 percent) compared with less than 40 percent in the general population had income from investments (interest, dividends, and rent). Perhaps less dramatic, a higher proportion of CCRC residents (more than 95 percent) had income from Social Security, a higher percentage than found in the general population (81 percent).

Notwithstanding inflation, which might account for a small amount of the difference, the economic status of CCRC apartment dwellers 75 years of age and older can be seen to be much higher than that of the total population. The recent residents were the richest, with a median annual income in 1986 between $30,000 and $40,000. The median of the longer-stay residents was between $20,000 and $30,000. In 1984, the national median household income of persons 75 years of age and older was under $20,000. Indeed, the difference in economic status between the national and CCRC populations is clearly illustrated by a comparison of the national percent below the poverty line with estimates made for the CCRC samples. None of the recent and very few (0.01 percent) of the longer-stay CCRC residents older than 75 years had household incomes below the poverty threshold (all of these persons lived alone). According to the SSA, as many as 17.7 percent of this age group fell below the poverty threshold in 1984 (U.S. DHHS SSA 1985). In 1980, 41.8 percent of this age group nationally had household incomes of at least twice the poverty level. In contrast, 98 percent of the recent and 96 percent of the longer-stay residents had incomes of at least twice the poverty level.

Age-Stratified Comparisons

CCRC Residents and Massachusetts Elderly Persons. It is possible that differential age distributions might account at least in part for other demographic differences observed between the overall samples of recent and longer-stay residents (e.g., in the percents female, married, widowed, and living alone in the CCRC). Some of the apparent demographic differences between people 75 years of age and older nationally and CCRC residents in this age group might also be explained, at least in part, by uneven age distributions within this category.

The final section of this chapter presents findings, by age group, from the comparisons of demographic, health and functional status, and miscellaneous other variables across CCRC recent residents, longer-stay residents, and Massachusetts elderly people and of the separate comparisons between CCRC recent and longer-term residents. These age-stratified findings shed light on this issue, providing a more meaningful context to the findings presented in subsequent chapters. In addition, although by no means definitive since we have limited comparable data pertaining to the characteristics of the longer-stay residents at entrance, age-stratified comparisons in a variety of domains between the samples of recent and longer-stay CCRC residents can provide insights as to similarities and potential changes in the types of persons entering CCRCs.

Demographic Characteristics. Comparisons were made regarding the percent with each of the following characteristics: female; lives alone (by self); four marital status variables (married, widowed, divorced/separated, and never married); racial identification variables (white, Hispanic, and foreign born); educational status variables (less than high school, high school, some college, college graduate); seven economic status variables [currently employed full/part time; income from personal investments; income from Social Security; annual income (greater than $20,000, $20,001 through $30,000, $30,001 through $50,000, and more than $50,000); Medicaid recipient; household income below the poverty level; and household income at least twice the poverty level]. This information is shown in Table 1.3.

Whereas few significant differences (at the 0.05 level) by age group were found between the CCRC samples of recent and longer-stay CCRC residents (70 through 74 years, 75 through 79 years, 80 through 84 years, and 85 years and older), the same could not be said for the three-way comparisons among Massachusetts elderly persons and the CCRC recent and longer-term residents. Of CCRC residents 70 years of age and older, recent and longer-stay residents in the youngest of these age groups (persons between 70 and 74 years) were most similar, with only one significant difference (e.g., educational status). Although educational status did not significantly differentiate recent and longer-stay residents in the older age groups, longer-stay residents tended to be better educated than the recent residents in the age group 70 through 74 years. Fewer college graduates were found among the recent (53 percent)

Table 1.3 Demographic characteristics of recent and longer-stay CCRC residents and Massachusetts (MA) sample, by age group

	70–74 years old			75–79 years old			80–84 years old			85+ years old		
	Recent (N=109)	Longer-stay (N=88)	MA (N=496)	Recent (N=165)	Longer-stay (N=285)	MA (N=444)	Recent (N=183)	Longer-stay (N=465)	MA (N=311)	Recent (N=100)	Longer-stay (N=575)	MA (N=196)
	%	%	%	%	%	%	%	%	%	%	%	%
Female	70.6	75.0	61.9	69.1	80.4#	56.5	65.6	78.5#	61.0	69.0	76.5	70.7+
Marital status												
Married	54.1	51.1	58.6+	60.6	44.9#	36.2	47.0	34.4#	36.5	38.0	23.8#	19.9
Widowed	30.3	28.4	31.3+	29.7	38.2	46.6	47.5	51.2	54.2+	57.0	62.6	72.4
Divorced/separated	3.7	4.5	4.3+	4.2	1.8	4.5+	2.7	1.7	3.0+	1.0	2.1	0.6+
Never married	11.9	16.0	5.8	5.5	15.1#	12.6	2.7	12.7#	6.3	4.0	11.5#	7.1
Lives alone (by self)	44.0	51.1	30.6	33.9	54.3#	43.9	53.0	65.4#	46.2	61.0	75.0#	46.9
Children nearby	34.9	28.3	71.8	30.4	21.5#	54.6	34.4	25.1#	65.7	42.0	29.6#	69.3
Race/ethnicity												
White	99.1	100.0	84.8	98.8	99.6	92.4	98.4	98.7	89.2	98.4	98.7	89.2
Hispanic	0.9	0.0	3.0+	0.0	0.0	0.2+	1.6	0.4	0.5+	0.0	0.5	0.3+
Foreign born	2.8	2.3	4.9+	4.8	6.3	6.6+	3.8	7.1	14.7	3.8	7.1	14.7

Educational status												
Less than high school	8.3	2.3	59.4	10.3	7.4	65.1	10.4	9.2	68.8	22.0	12.7	78.8
High school	18.3	10.2#	26.6	20.0	15.4	13.4	15.3	13.8	14.6	15.0	18.1	10.0
Some college	20.2	13.6	8.1	24.2	25.3	10.9	28.4	20.9	6.7	17.0	23.0	4.0
College graduate	53.2	73.9	5.9	45.5	51.9	10.7	45.9	56.1	9.1	46.0	46.3	5.5
Economic status												
Currently employed	4.6	11.4	17.6	3.0	3.2	11.0	1.6	1.9	5.5	3.0	2.4	1.0+
Income from												
Personal investments	96.3	98.9	63.7	98.8	95.8	69.2	94.0	95.7	65.5	96.0	92.2	59.9
Social Security	97.2	98.9	95.7+	97.6	96.8	94.7+	94.5	94.6	93.7+	97.0	94.6	90.0
Medicaid recipient	0.9	1.1	6.7	0.6	0.0	13.6	1.6	0.9	7.8	2.0	0.7	12.3
Annual income[a]												
Less than $20,000	19.3	20.5	62.0	18.8	22.5	65.4	15.3	23.5	72.9	22.0	26.1	72.8
$20,001–$30,000	31.2	34.1	21.6	28.5	30.5	15.3	30.1	31.3	14.9	30.0	28.2	18.5
$30,001–$50,000	30.3	25.0	14.5	29.1	28.0	17.5	34.4	28.2	11.1	35.0	32.9	8.1
Over $50,000	19.3	20.5	1.8	23.6	18.9	1.9	20.2	17.0	0.6	13.0	12.9	0.0
Below poverty level[a]	0.0	0.0	8.4	0.0	0.0	14.5	0.0	0.0	20.0	0.0	0.0	28.2
Twice over poverty level[a]	97.1	100.0	46.3	100.0	95.7	27.6	99.9	97.6	27.6	93.3	95.8	23.6

Note. All differences between the CCRC samples and the MA sample are statistically significant (at the 0.05 probability level) except where are marked with a +, noted in each case, directly after the Massachusetts sample percentage. No significant differences occur between recent (of less than one year) CCRC residents and longer-stay (one year or more) residents except where marked with a #, noted directly after the longer-stay CCRC percentage.

[a]Because of lack of detailed data, CCRC estimates were derived from follow-up data.

than the longer-stay (74 percent) residents, and more of the recent than longer-stay residents had less than a high school education (8 percent compared with 2 percent, respectively).

The CCRC residents 70 through 74 years of age were also most similar to their age counterparts in the Massachusetts population, but even for this age group, significant differences were found across the Massachusetts residents and the two CCRC samples in more than two thirds of the comparisons. No differences were found in the across-sample comparisons in the percents Hispanic, foreign born, with income from Social Security, or, except for the never married, in any of the other marital status categories. Similarities persisted in the proportion of Hispanics in all age groups and in the proportion with income from Social Security in all but the 85 and older age group.

Reflecting their distribution in the national population in general, almost all of the residents in each of the CCRC samples were white. The proportions white were significantly higher for the CCRC apartment dwellers than for the Massachusetts community population in each of the four age groups.

As might be expected, the majority were female in all three samples and in all age groups. At the same time, except for the oldest age group (persons 85 years and older), significant differences in the proportion female were found across the elderly Massachusetts residents and CCRC samples. In the two groups between 75 and 84 years of age, higher proportions of CCRC residents were female, with significantly higher proportions in the longer-stay than in the recent resident samples.

Although in the Massachusetts samples a majority in each of the four age groups had children nearby, only a small number of CCRC residents, recent or longer-stay, had children nearby. As might be expected, the percent of the population in the widowed category rose for the most part with age; in the 85 and older age category, the majority were widowed — 57 percent of the recent CCRC residents, 63 percent of the CCRC residents of a year or more, and as many as 72 percent of the Massachusetts sample. The majority in each of the samples under 75 were married, with no significant differences among CCRC and Massachusetts residents. However, several differences between recent and longer-stay CCRC residents in the older age groups were conceptually related to differences found in marital status. Specifically, from ages 75 on,

▪   more recent than longer-stay CCRC or traditional-community residents were still married, whereas more longer-stay than recent CCRC or traditional-community residents were never married;

- correspondingly, in each of the age groups, significantly more of the longer-stay residents lived alone;
- significantly fewer of the longer-stay than recent residents had children within a one-hour drive;
- CCRC residents were consistently better educated and economically better off than their age peers in the Massachusetts samples. Only a very few in any of the samples were gainfully employed, but, up to the age of 85, more of the Massachusetts than the CCRC residents were in this category.

Health and Functional Status. Fifteen variables representing health conditions and key areas of functional status — basic activities of daily living, instrumental activities of daily living, mobility, and mental functioning — were selected for this analysis. These were: having one or more medical conditions; eleven variables regarding whether help was needed with personal and instrumental activities of daily living (personal care; dressing; getting out of a chair; preparing bath; managing medications; preparing meals; light housework; heavy housekeeping and chores such as hanging curtains; taking out the garbage; shopping or performing small errands; and transportation); and three variables regarding mobility, specifically the ability to climb stairs, walk a half-mile, walk twenty feet (see Table 1.4).

When CCRC and traditional-community Massachusetts residents were compared by age category on this series of health and functional status characteristics, the subsamples between 70 and 74 years of age (the youngest of the four age groups) were most similar. No significant differences on any of these variables were found in this age group between recent residents and the longer-stay CCRC residents, and significant differences across the CCRC and Massachusetts subsamples occurred in only four instances. Older persons outside the CCRC needed help with taking out the garbage, shopping and performing small errands, transportation, and walking a half-mile. In each case, CCRC residents (both recent and longer-term residents) had better functional status than their age counterparts in the Massachusetts community. In fact, for each of these four variables this finding persisted in all of the age groups.

No differences were found in health and functional status between recent and longer-stay CCRC residents in the age group 75 through 79 years. There were a few differences between recent and longer-stay CCRC residents in the two oldest age groups, generally indicating that functionally the longer-stay residents were in slightly worse shape than

Table 1.4 Comparisons between selected baseline health and functional status characteristics of recent and longer-stay CCRC residents and the Massachusetts (MA) elderly, by age group

	70–74 years old			75–79 years old			80–84 years old			85+ years old		
	Recent (N = 109)	Longer-stay (N = 88)	MA (N = 496)	Recent (N = 165)	Longer-stay (N = 285)	MA (N = 444)	Recent (N = 183)	Longer-stay (N = 465)	MA (N = 311)	Recent (N = 100)	Longer-stay (N = 575)	MA (N = 196)
	%	%	%	%	%	%	%	%	%	%	%	%
Health												
1+ Medical problems[a]	85.3	86.4	82.6+	92.7	92.6	83.6	86.9	92.9	85.5	93.0	92.2	90.6+
Physical functioning												
Needs help with												
Personal care	0.0	1.1	3.7+	3.6	2.8	4.4+	1.6	3.7	8.6	3.0	8.2	17.1
Dressing	3.7	9.1	3.6+	7.9	7.4	1.6	4.4	6.2	8.7+	4.0	8.9	11.6+
Getting out of chair	0.0	1.1	2.0+	0.0	1.4	1.6+	0.0	1.3	3.2+	0.0	3.8	7.7+
Preparing bath	0.0	2.3	7.1+	4.2	2.5	5.7+	1.6	4.5	8.6	2.0	8.0#	18.3
Managing medications	0.0	1.1	3.5+	3.0	1.8	1.8+	3.8	1.9	6.5+	6.0	6.8	15.1
Preparing meals	5.5	4.5	7.9+	7.9	4.9	8.0+	7.9	6.9	16.4	14.0	13.9	26.1
Light housework	7.4	12.5	14.2+	10.9	10.2	12.1+	12.0	12.9	28.3	20.0	23.5	46.6
Heavy cleaning/chores	32.1	43.2	33.7+	41.3	46.3	36.5	51.9	61.3#	51.9	62.0	71.5	67.3+
Taking out garbage	6.4	8.0	14.5	10.9	7.8	15.0	8.1	8.0	24.7	10.1	16.4	41.2
Shopping/errands	3.7	8.0	19.7	9.1	6.7	21.0	7.1	9.5	37.8	16.0	22.3	57.5
Transportation	1.8	5.7	16.3	4.8	7.0	18.4	10.4	10.1	34.5	23.0	18.3	57.7
Mobility: able to												
Climb stairs	95.4	94.3	89.7+	94.5	91.9	91.0+	96.7	90.3#	87.4	91.8	82.8#	76.5
Walk ½ mile	92.4	87.2	80.9	90.0	88.2	73.3	91.0	83.2#	54.9	77.3	69.2	35.8
Walk 20 feet	97.2	96.6	92.9+	97.0	97.5	89.5	97.8	96.3	87.2	97.0	92.0	77.6

Note. All differences between the CCRC samples and the MA sample were statistically significant (at the 0.05 probability level) except where marked with a +, noted in each case, directly after the Massachusetts sample percentage. No significant differences occurred between recent (of less than one year) CCRC residents and longer-stay (of one year or more) residents except where marked with a #, noted directly after the longer-stay CCRC percentage.

[a]One or more of the following conditions: arthritis; high blood pressure; heart problem; diabetes; stroke; other neurological, cancer, orthopedic, emphysema or other pulmonary condition; circulatory/vascular problems.

the more recent residents. Significantly more of the longer-stay than recent residents who were 80 through 84 years old said that they needed help with heavy cleaning and chores, and, although the majority had no problems in these areas, fewer of the longer-stay residents claimed that they were able to climb stairs or walk a half-mile. In the 85 and older age group, only a small proportion of the residents had such problems, but significantly fewer of the longer-stay residents in this age group said that they were able to climb stairs, and more said that they needed help with bathing.

The Massachusetts sample fared better than the CCRC age group subsamples in a few instances, found only in comparisons of the middle two age groups (75 through 79 and 80 through 84 years). Although a large majority of all four age groups suffered from one or more medical problems, this was the case for significantly fewer of the Massachusetts community residents in these two age groups. Also, similar to the proportion of recent CCRC residents needing such help, fewer of the Massachusetts than the longer-stay CCRC residents between 80 and 84 years of age needed help with heavy cleaning/chores.

In general, however, differences across the three samples within each age group favored the CCRC populations. Furthermore, the number of such differences increased by age group, with differences found for as few as 25 percent of the variables across the samples in the 70 through 74 year group to as many as 69 percent in the 85 and older age group.

Nevertheless, Massachusetts and CCRC residents were similar in several respects. For example, a large majority (more than 80 percent) in each subsample within each age group had one or more medical problems. In contrast, for functional status variables, a majority, often a large majority, in each of these samples was functionally intact. These people did not need help with various types of personal and instrumental activities of daily living, and they were mobile.

Activities and Miscellaneous Other Variables. The final set of age-stratified comparisons across the CCRC and Massachusetts samples and between the recent and longer-stay CCRC residents included the following (Table 1.5):

- whether or not the sample member usually went out of the house (or building, if in an apartment) more than one day a week;
- how much time (from little to considerable) the sample member spent chatting on the phone or visiting in person with friends;
- how much time the sample member spent chatting on the phone or visiting in person with family members;

Table 1.5 Baseline comparisons across recent and longer-stay CCRC residents and Massachusetts (MA) elderly regarding decision making, activities, informal support, and support-related concerns, by age group

	70–74 years old			75–79 years old			80–84 years old			85+ years old		
	Recent (N=109)	Longer-stay (N=88)	MA (N=496)	Recent (N=165)	Longer-stay (N=285)	MA (N=444)	Recent (N=183)	Longer-stay (N=465)	MA (N=311)	Recent (N=100)	Longer-stay (N=575)	MA (N=196)
	%	%	%	%	%	%	%	%	%	%	%	%
Activities/social interactions												
Venture out of house more than once a week	100.0	98.9	94.9+	98.2	97.2	91.8	98.4	95.1	85.4	96.0	91.8	73.9
Time spent visiting/phoning friends												
Little	28.4	18.2	28.7	30.3	18.6	31.8	31.3	22.4	34.3	41.0	24.2	49.2
Some	33.9	40.9	28.8+	38.8	38.6#	30.4	46.7	38.3#	32.2	33.0	41.3#	23.6
Considerable	37.6	40.9	42.5	30.9	42.8	37.8	22.0	39.4	33.6	26.0	34.5	27.1
Time spent visiting/phoning family												
Little	40.4	35.2	13.5	38.8	41.1	15.0	34.3	41.3	15.9	36.0	43.4	16.2
Some	25.7	29.5	22.7	32.7	28.8	22.6	35.4	29.7	26.2	36.0	29.6	28.9
Considerable	34.9	45.3	63.8	28.5	30.1	62.4	30.3	29.0	57.9	28.0	27.0	54.1

	100.0	98.9	97.7+	98.2	98.2	96.8+	95.6	98.1	93.8	95.0	94.9	90.5+
Independence												
Makes own decisions	100.0	98.9	97.7+	98.2	98.2	96.8+	95.6	98.1	93.8	95.0	94.9	90.5+
If unable to care for themselves physically, where should old persons live?[a]												
Nursing home	8.0	13.3	21.3	10.5	13.2	17.5+	9.2	12.2	17.6	11.6	9.1	16.5
Child/relative	1.0	2.4	11.8	3.2	1.9	6.6	2.9	1.8	16.6	7.5	3.4	26.8
Own home with help[b]	85.0	78.3	39.4	79.7	82.3	34.8	84.4	81.9	38.9	79.6	82.7	31.8
Doesn't want to think about it	3.0	3.6	27.2	3.8	1.5	40.1	2.3	1.8	25.9	2.2	2.8	24.2
Other[c]	3.0	2.4	0.3+	2.5	1.1	1.0+	1.2	2.3	1.0+	0.0	2.0	0.7+
Informal supports												
Child	55.0	38.6#	69.7	52.7	36.1#	55.6	56.8	44.1#	65.4	62.0	47.0#	70.1
Friend	34.9	45.5	22.2	42.4	48.4	24.2	43.2	47.7	24.2	45.0	38.8	23.9

Note. All differences between the CCRC samples and the MA sample were statistically significant (at the 0.05 probability level) except where marked with a +, noted in each case directly after the Massachusetts sample percentage. No significant differences occurred between recent (of less than one year) CCRC residents and longer-stay (of one year or more) residents except where marked with a #, noted directly after the two CCRC data columns.

[a] Sample members unable to care for themselves who were living in the community in the home of a child and not asked this question were classified as if they had responded *with children*; those in this category who were living in their own home with spouse as caretaker were classified as if they had responded *at home with help*.

[b] Included the following responses: their own home; CCRC or retirement community; or housing for the elderly.

[c] Included responses such as the following: better off dead; commit suicide; personal/foster home care (licensed and unlicensed).

- whether or not a child (including in-laws) was among those named (of up to four persons) who helped the most or who the sample member felt could be most relied upon to help if needed;
- whether or not a friend was among those who helped the most or who the sample member felt could be relied upon to help if needed;
- whether, in general, the sample member made decisions alone (or with a spouse) as opposed to doing what others thought best or letting others make their decisions (including spouse, other family, or friends);
- attitudes as to where people should live when they reach old age and are unable to care for themselves physically.

Separate statistical analyses were conducted for a series of key responses to this last question, categorized as follows: nursing home; child or other relative; a category labeled *own home with help* (which also included responses indicating CCRC/retirement community and specialized housing for elderly people); a denial category (did not want to think about it and/or had not thought about it previously); and *other* as a catch-all for the few remaining responses.

Although many differences were found between Massachusetts and CCRC samples in each of these age groups, there were few significant differences between recent and longer-stay residents. In the 70 through 79 year age groups, the separate comparisons of recent and longer-stay CCRC residents revealed only one variance: recent residents were more likely to name a child as a key helper. This difference was found consistently in the remaining age group comparisons as well. There was only one other distinction between recent and longer-stay residents in the remaining age groups: in each of these age-stratified comparisons, longer-stay CCRC residents spent more time than recent residents in visiting and phoning friends. On both these variables, recent residents of 75 years of age and older resembled their age peers in the Massachusetts community rather than the longer-stay residents.

The Massachusetts and CCRC subsamples in the youngest age category, 70 through 74 years of age, were the most similar. No significant difference across the samples was observed in whether the sample members ventured out of the house more than once a week; time spent visiting or chatting with friends by phone; and whether they made their own decisions. In only one age group, for persons between 80 and 84 years, was a significant across-sample difference found in decision making (with CCRC residents, particularly the longer-term residents, more likely to make their own decisions). Significant across-sample differences for venturing out of the house and for time spent visiting or chatting with friends, however, were found in each of the three older age groups, even though a large majority in all samples, regardless of age group, said they left the house more than once a week and spent some or considerable time interacting with friends. In each of the three older age groups, fewer Massachusetts community residents than either recent or longer-stay CCRC residents went out more than once a week, and, similar to the recent CCRC residents, they tended to spend less time visiting or chatting with friends than did the longer-stay CCRC residents.

A majority in all samples, regardless of age category, said they spent some or considerable time interacting with family members. Nevertheless, in each of the age-stratified comparisons, the Massachusetts sample members were likely to spend more time interacting with family members than either the recent or longer-stay CCRC residents. Significant differences in favor of the Massachusetts samples were also found in each of the separate age group comparisons for another somewhat related variable — whether a child was named as a key helper. Like the CCRC recent residents, a majority of Massachusetts residents named at least one child as a key informal helper, significantly more than the longer-stay residents. In no instance did a majority of persons name a friend as a key helper, but in this case, in each of the age-stratified comparisons, significantly fewer Massachusetts than CCRC residents, recent or longer-stay, named a friend among those in the informal system who provided the most help or could be relied upon to provide such help.

Finally, with few exceptions, there were significant differences between Massachusetts and CCRC residents in their opinions as to where people should live when they reach old age and are unable to care for themselves physically. In each age group, more than three quarters of CCRC residents, both recent and longer-stay, compared with a minority (fewer than 40 percent) of elderly Massachusetts residents, chose the *own home with help* option.

Only small minorities in each of the age-stratified samples thought that older persons unable to care for themselves physically should live in a nursing home (between 8 and 21 percent) or that they should live with children or other family members (between 1 and 27 percent). However, except for the age group between 75 and 79 years of age, significantly more of the Massachusetts sample responded *nursing home*, and significantly more in all four of the age categories chose this response.

Significant differences were found consistently in the age-stratified comparisons between CCRC and Massachusetts residents in the proportions responding that they never thought about this issue and/or they did not want to think about it. In the total sample, fewer than than 4 percent in any of the CCRC samples expressed this, but in the Massachusetts samples, between 24 percent (85 years of age and older) and 40 percent (between 75 and 79 years of age) did so.

Conclusions and Insights
Age-Stratified Comparisons

By and large, the age-stratified comparisons do not dramatically change the study's conclusions about the types of persons who are CCRC residents. Both recent and longer-stay CCRC residents in the three age-stratified groups 75 years and older (75 through 79, 80 through 84, and 85 years and older) remain very different demographically from their age group peers in the traditional community. Regardless of age group or how recent the CCRC entrance, in general CCRCs serve white, well-educated, economically solvent segments of the elderly population. At the same time, even among populations 75 years of age and older, CCRC residents are on average older than their counterparts in the community. Only a very small minority in any of the samples were gainfully employed, but, at least up to the age of 85, more of the Massachusetts than the CCRC residents were in this category. Similarly, although the majority in all groups were female, except for age 85 and older, significantly more CCRC than Massachusetts community residents in each age group were women. Just as in the descriptive differences found between CCRC residents and their age peers in the national population, CCRC longer-stay residents in these three age groups tended to be more like the community in the percentages married and widowed than were recent residents. However, at least in the groups 80 years of age and older, they were more like the recent residents in the percentages never married. In general, larger proportions of the CCRC residents lived alone.

Although many of the across-sample differences in the age-stratified comparisons of CCRC and Massachusetts samples of persons 75 years and older persisted even in the younger age group, the Massachusetts and CCRC populations 70 through 74 years of age tended to be most similar. This was the case regarding demographic variables as well as others. In general, in health and functional status and in activities and other miscellaneous quality-of-life variables, the number of significant differences also increased by age group.

These differences were often but not always in favor of the CCRC samples. As demonstrated by the recent residents in particular but also by the longer-stay residents, the CCRC residents were drawn from better functioning segments of the elderly population. Yet fewer elderly Massachusetts residents than longer-stay CCRC residents between the ages of 75 and 84 years reported having medical problems or needing help with heavy cleaning or chores.

Differences in expectations and the actual role of the informal system in addressing the needs of CCRC and traditional-community residents are suggested by a combination of a number of demographic findings. For one, elderly Massachusetts residents were more likely to have children nearby. In addition, in the older groups (when concerns about possible deteriorating health might become more relevant), Massachusetts residents were less likely to live alone even though, compared with the CCRC samples, they were less or equally likely to be married. As first suggested in the comparisons of CCRC residents 75 years of age and older with their age peers nationally, it does seem that joining the CCRC might be taking the place of the informal system in giving residence and support services to elderly people who become widowed and frail.

Several findings regarding activities and informal supports lend further support to this insight. From age 75 and beyond, the elderly Massachusetts residents spent more time visiting and phoning their family, and they were more likely than the CCRC residents to have children in their informal support system. On the other hand, the CCRC residents in each age category were likely to spend more time visiting and phoning friends than were the Massachusetts sample. They were also more likely than Massachusetts sample in each of the age groups to name a friend as a key helper. Once again, particularly in light of the finding regarding the smaller proportions of CCRC residents with children in this role, it would seem that the informal support system of CCRC residents can be expected to be different — playing a qualitatively more minor role — in addressing their supportive service needs. This, in fact, might be a goal of CCRC residents: to maintain more independence and self-reliance by planning for access to formal services should assistance with activities of daily living be needed.

In fact, the educational status and occupation of the CCRC residents pointed to planning and independence as key life-style descriptors of them. Both recent and longer-stay CCRC residents tended to be highly educated, with a large majority completing at least one or more years of college — a relatively rare phenomenon for this age group, particularly for women. Furthermore, even though females predominated in the CCRC samples, a large majority of the CCRC residents had been in the labor force most of their lives. Many of the CCRC residents, including the female population, were professionals, proprietors, and managers — positions that generally have planning and decision-making responsibilities. Experience in such positions in many ways can be expected to reinforce and enhance the ability to plan and be self-reliant.

The responses of the CCRC subsamples compared with Massachusetts samples to the question of where a frail elderly person should live are also indicative of greater willingness to face and plan for issues that might be seen as unpleasant (a planning perspective) and of a greater inclination for an independent life style. More CCRC than Massachusetts residents in each age group chose an independent living option; more favored staying in one's home with help, and fewer favored entering a nursing home. It is, of course, possible that some of the few persons who selected a CCRC for this question and thus were classified in the own-home-with-help category, regarded CCRCs as a mechanism for aging in place, including the possibility of transfer to a CCRC health center (nursing home) when necessary. In any event, a greater willingness on the part of the Massachusetts sample to depend on family members was exhibited by the number in each age group who said they would move in with a child or some other relative when those already living with family members were counted as part of the group who chose this option. What was perhaps most interesting, although perhaps to be expected considering the long-term care planning features of a CCRC, a much larger proportion of the Massachusetts sample than the CCRC residents in each age group said they never thought about it and/or did not want to think about it. Very few CCRC residents responded this way, but about one quarter or more of the Massachusetts sample in each of the age categories did so.

Recent and Longer-Stay CCRC Residents

The age-stratified comparisons of recent and longer-stay residents revealed few differences, regardless of age category. As in the across-sample comparisons, the younger the age group, the fewer differences found.

In the categories concerning physical functioning, the few differences between recent and longer-stay residents in the older age groups were, perhaps, to be expected. That recent residents in the two oldest age categories enjoyed somewhat better functional status is understandable because of the intake policies of CCRCs that are fiscally responsible in whole or part for providing long-term care services. For economic reasons alone, CCRCs need to ensure that new residents will not need nursing home care for a reasonable length of time.

Although in general there seems to be little change in the types of residents joining a CCRC, some differences suggest that the concept of the CCRC is spreading to a broader segment of the population. In particular, this conclusion is indicated by the larger percentages of recent than longer-stay residents in the three older age groups who are married and not living alone at entrance, have children nearby, and who name a child as a key helper in their informal support systems.

The slightly lower educational status of the two youngest groups of recent residents suggests that the concept is broadening slightly in this area as well. However, older persons joining the CCRC have as much education as their counterparts among longer-stay residents. Not surprising, therefore, differences found in educational achievement in the two younger age categories did not hold for the samples as a whole. Furthermore, the average age of recent residents was actually higher than the average age at entrance of the longer-stay residents (78.1 and 76.7 years of age, respectively). Therefore, even if younger persons entering the CCRC continue to include larger proportions with less educational attainment, the characteristics of the overall populations of recent and longer-stay residents are not likely to be affected in this regard.

There was one other age-stratified finding that differed from the overall comparisons of recent and longer-stay residents. Specifically, even though recent residents were likely to have higher incomes than those who had been in the CCRC for a year or more, no such differences were significant in the age-stratified comparisons of economic status. This suggests that economic differences within each age group were small but cumulative.

Finally, there was a relatively consistent difference that suggested the possible influence that living in a CCRC for a longer period of time had on developing friendships. Except for the age group of 70 through 74 years, longer-stay residents spent significantly more time visiting or phoning friends than did the recent residents. Although not statistically significant, the difference was in the same direction for the group of 70- through 74-year-olds as well.

TWO

Extended and Limited CCRCs: Residents' Background Characteristics and Reasons for Entrance

This chapter focuses on similarities and differences in background characteristics and the reasons residents gave for moving into a CCRC. In Chapter 1 we differentiated extended and limited CCRCs based upon their degree of protection against unanticipated future expenditures for nursing home care. Extended CCRCs provide such care on a virtually unlimited basis at little or no extra cost to the resident, except for the additional meals not ordinarily provided by the monthly fee. Facilities providing less financial protection against the high costs of nursing home care are considered limited CCRCs, whether they provide this type of care for a full or discounted fee-for-service. This distinction suggests the possibility that these two types of CCRC might attract different sorts of persons as well as the possibility that the experience of residents within these facilities might differ.

Other CCRC structural and contract characteristics that relate to the facility's ambiance and cost considerations may differ in extended and limited CCRCs, for example, size, occupancy rates, proportion of nursing home beds to apartments, the entrance and monthly fees charged, and services included in these fees. Differences in these characteristics can also be expected to impact on attractiveness to, and the experience of, residents in these two types of CCRC.

The first part of this chapter describes and compares nine extended CCRCs with ten limited CCRCs. A picture of similarities and differences in organizational features between the two CCRC types can provide further insights as to the differences that might be found between the resident populations.

In the next part, the residents of extended and limited CCRCs are first compared on selected characteristics at the time of entrance. Similarities and differences in baseline characteristics of the two samples when they were first interviewed are then compared. These comparisons focus on social, health/functional status, and economic variables that, particularly for longer-stay residents, may have changed since entrance and theoretically influenced their selective recall about why they joined the CCRC. The final part of this chapter compares the residents' reasons for entering a CRCC.

A Comparison of Extended and Limited CCRC Facility Characteristics
Data Sources and Analyses

We derived our data for comparing nine extended CCRCs with ten limited CCRCs from two sources: an organizational questionnaire filled out by administrators (or their designees); and an analysis of the content of facility contracts offered by the two types of CCRC. We reviewed the information that was collected systematically from these two sources, focusing on organizational features that may have made a difference in facility ambiance and costs to persons considering a CCRC, aside from the basis for classification as extended or limited CCRCs. Because of the small number of CCRCs in the study, comparisons among sample groups are descriptive in nature.

We compared the following organizational characteristics of CCRCs: religious affiliation, number of years in operation, size, occupancy, number of health care beds, entrance fee, and monthly fee. For descriptions of the comprehensiveness of services that were specifically included in the monthly fees and guaranteed by the CCRC contracts we analyzed the contracts and used data culled from the organizational questionnaire which pertained to supportive services. Contracts provided by the CCRCs generally backed up what was reported in the organizational questionnaire.

We should note that the number of contracts tended to vary with the number of years that the CCRC had been in operation. Six of the newest facilities have had only one contract, and one facility, in existence since 1961, has had at least ten. However, contract provisions for each of the nineteen CCRCs remained relatively constant over time in terms of protection against unanticipated nursing home costs. In other words, according to our definitions, facilities that had offered extended type contracts when they began operation continued to offer such contracts, and the same held true for facilities offering limited type contracts. Contractual changes were most likely to include increases in fees or a change in refund policy.

Extended and Limited CCRC Characteristics

The nine CCRCs in our study which offered extended contracts included four of the five Pennsylvania sites, two of the four Arizona sites, two of the five California sites, and one of the five Florida sites. Reflecting the vast majority of CCRCs in operation, all nineteen of these facilities, limited and extended, were nonprofit.

Religious Affiliation. None of the study CCRCs claimed that religious identification was used as a criterion of acceptance or rejection of applicants. Nevertheless, the majority of both the limited and extended CCRCs — six of the nine extended and eight of the ten limited CCRCs — reported some sort of relationship with a religious organization (e.g., with 20 percent or more of the board members connected to the religious organization). However, only two of the extended and one of the limited CCRCs with affiliations noted that the religious organization assumed any financial liability for the CCRC.

Size. The extended CCRCs were, on average, considerably larger than the limited CCRCs. The mean number of independent living units (ILUs, hereinafter usually referred to as apartments) in the former was 340 (ranging from 181 to 511 apartments) and in the latter 224 (ranging from 100 to 329 apartments).

Years in Operation. One limited CCRC had its roots in the last century (in 1986 it had been in operation for ninety-six years). Otherwise, the range in years of operation for the extended and limited CCRCs in our study was roughly similar — from two to twenty-two years (an average of 9.6) for the nine remaining limited facilities and from two to twenty-four years (with an average of 11.2 years) for the nine extended CCRCs.[1]

Occupancy. The occupancy rates of both types of CCRC were high. The extended CCRCs had a higher mean rate (99 percent) of occupancy, ranging from a low of 92 percent for one facility to a high of 100 percent for seven. In the limited CCRCs the mean rate was 90 percent, ranging from a low of 75 percent for one facility to a high of 100 percent for three. There appeared to be no correlation between occupancy rate and the number of years of operation. For example, the fully occupied limited facilities included the facility in existence for ninety-six years, one facility in operation for seven years, and another for twenty-two years. Of the two limited facilities with occupancy rates under 80 percent, the one with the lowest rate had been in operation for twenty-two years and the second (78 percent occupied) for only seven years.

1. Interestingly, CCRCs in operation for more than ten years had lower residential unit and health center costs per day than the newer CCRCs.

Health Care Beds and Certification Status. Only two of the nine extended compared with seven of the ten limited CCRCs had personal care or assisted living units. There was more similarity in the ratio of nursing home beds to apartments. For example, limited CCRCs had a ratio of from 0.2 to 0.8 nursing home beds to one apartment, with a mean ratio of 0.34; the ratios for extended CCRCs ranged from 0.15 to 0.85, with a mean of 0.37. The nursing home beds in the majority of both types of CCRC were Medicare certified, some of which had Medicaid certification as well. Specifically, three of the nine extended CCRCs were both Medicare and Medicaid certified, four were Medicare certified only, and two had neither Medicaid nor Medicare certification. Of the ten limited CCRCs, four had both Medicare and Medicaid certification, an additional three had Medicare certification only, and three were neither Medicare nor Medicaid certified.[2]

Services Included in the Monthly Fee. Both the extended and limited CCRCs offered many amenities and activity programs, with limited type facilities offering at least as many as the extended CCRCs. Although somewhat more so in the extended CCRCs, almost all included a package of supportive services to their apartment-dwelling residents at no additional cost above the monthly fee. All of the extended and eight of the limited CCRCs included one or more meals in the monthly fee. Also, all extended and seven of limited included light housekeeping. One of the two limited CCRCs not including light housekeeping did include window washing as part of the monthly fee. Contracts for five of the extended facilities also referred to a broad range of community health services: prescription medicines, hospitalization, medical and surgical services, physician services, and temporary nursing care in a skilled nursing unit. However, coverage was limited to services provided by medical and nursing staff affiliated with, or referred by, the CCRC. Contracts also required that the resident purchase all public forms of health insurance for which they were eligible, specifically Medicare Parts A and B and the Blue Cross 65 Special Plan.

Of the nine extended CCRCs, the five that provided the broad package of community health care services to apartment dwellers at no additional cost also offered residents the most comprehensive service packages at no additional cost. Of these sites, four facilities included three meals a day, although one permitted residents to choose only the

2. Considering all of the facilities, with and without Medicare and Medicaid certification, the cost of care provided in a CCRC health center appeared to be comparable to the private-pay rate for nursing home care in the economy at large.

main meal in the dining room and have the monthly fee reduced accordingly; the fifth CCRC offered residents the option of including one to three meals in the monthly fee. In addition to meals, housekeeping, and laundry, four facilities included scheduled transportation, two including transportation to medical appointments as well, and the fifth CCRC included transportation to medical appointments and to planned activities.

For three of the remaining four extended facilities, supportive services also included, at no cost above the monthly fee, one meal a day, housekeeping on a weekly or biweekly basis, flat laundry services, and scheduled transportation services and transportation to medical appointments. One of these three CCRCs also included transportation to planned activities. The fourth CCRC included in the monthly fee all of these services except transportation. In these CCRCs, residents who were transferred temporarily or permanently to the skilled nursing unit paid the cost of meals that were not included in the contract in addition to their monthly fee.

The most extensive community service packages provided as part of the monthly fee by limited CCRCs were similar to the last four extended CCRCs described above. Four of the ten limited CCRCs offered such packages. One included three meals a day, housekeeping, and laundry, but no transportation services, and residents paid the current private pay rate for nursing home care, whether the move from the ILU was temporary or permanent. Three facilities included one meal a day, housekeeping on a weekly or biweekly basis, flat laundry, and transportation — one with a robust transportation package (including regularly scheduled transportation and transportation to medical appointments and to planned activities) — and two facilities with regularly scheduled transportation and transportation to planned activities as well. Two of these three CCRCs provided coverage for ninety days per year in their skilled nursing units. (Note: Residents of these sites would not be reimbursed for Medicare-covered stays because the sites did not accept Medicare payments.) For stays beyond ninety days in a calendar year, the resident paid 100 percent of the market rate if the apartment was not released or 80 percent of the prevailing rate if the apartment was released. The third CCRC required payment for additional meals only when the move to the health center was temporary but payment according to a rate specified in the resident's contract when the move was permanent.

A fifth site included one meal a day, light housekeeping on a biweekly basis, and transportation to medical appointments and planned activities as well as regularly scheduled trips. Residents moving permanently into the nursing home might be charged less than the prevailing rate for a nursing home stay (the resident contract permitted the rate of reduction to fluctuate).

The monthly fee for the sixth limited CCRC included one meal a day, light housekeeping on a biweekly basis, and regularly scheduled transportation services. Residents of this CCRC paid the prevailing private rate for nursing home care.

Three of the remaining four limited CCRCs included only two services as part of the monthly fee. One CCRC included three meals a day and window washing on a biweekly basis. The second included a package of transportation services (scheduled, to medical appointments, and to planned activities) and one meal a day. The third facility included a similar package of transportation and light housekeeping on a monthly basis. The first of these three sites charged for additional meals only for temporary nursing home stays, but it charged a rate specified in the resident's contract when the move was permanent. A resident of the second site was allowed five days in the nursing home in a twelve-month period for only the cost of meals; after the apartment was released the resident had to pay the full cost of nursing home care. The third site accepted no Medicare, and residents would pay the full market rate for nursing home stays, regardless of whether the move was temporary or permanent.

The final limited CCRC had the least extensive service package. All services (including nursing home care) except transportation to planned activities were charged for on a fee-for-service basis.

Entrance and Monthly Fees. It can be seen that, in addition to the added protection against the high costs of a lengthy stay in a nursing home, extended CCRC residents enjoyed, on average, more community health and supportive services as part of their monthly fee. Correspondingly, the mean entrance and monthly fees of extended CCRCs were higher than those of limited CCRCs. For the extended CCRCs in our study, the mean entrance fee in 1986 for a one-bedroom apartment was $53,378 (ranging from $24,205 to $66,125), and the mean monthly fee was $979 (ranging from $710 to $1,321). The mean entrance fee for the limited CCRC one-bedroom apartment was $48,756 (ranging from $24,665 to $74,000), and the mean monthly fee was $677 (with a range of $296 to $950).

Of the nineteen CCRCs, the five that offered the most comprehensive health and service packages — all extended CCRCs — charged the highest *monthly* fees, but only two of the five communities with the highest *entrance* fees were extended CCRCs. Yet, the site with the lowest entrance fee was an extended CCRC. The remaining four of the five CCRCs with the lowest entrance fees, and all five with the lowest monthly fees, were limited CCRCs.

It should be noted that entry fees and monthly maintenance fees were related positively to the daily cost of CCRC living (which was found to be a little higher than noted in published data on the cost of general community living[3]). However, the relationship between the entry fee and cost was much stronger than between the monthly fee and cost. The entry and monthly fees themselves, however, were not statistically related.

Contractual Promises Regarding Subsidies. Although some residents may have left because of a reversal in economic status, none of the CCRCs reported asking a resident to leave for this reason. In fact, contracts of four of the extended and four of the limited CCRCs stated specifically that residents would not be terminated solely because of an inability to pay their monthly fee. Of the five remaining extended CCRCs, two required the resident to apply for all governmental benefits before they would subsidize the fee; one promised to apply the unamortized portion of the entrance fee before terminating the resident; one facility would review the situation and might agree to subsidize the resident; and the fifth made no mention of this issue in its contract. Of the five limited CCRCs with no specific guarantee, two would explore all means before discharging the resident; the third one required the resident to apply for benefits from governmental agencies; the fourth would allow the resident to draw upon any unamortized portion of entrance fee before being asked to leave; and the fifth included no mention of this situation in its contract.

The Study CCRCs: Conclusions and Insights

Although CCRCs in general have many characteristics in common, market forces have permitted or facilitated considerable variation in how continuing care is provided within and between limited and extended CCRCs. It is reasonable to expect that differences in potential costs associated with transfer to the CCRC nursing home, other cost issues (e.g., entrance and monthly fees and fees for supportive services) along with other organizational and environmental considerations that

---

3. Given the enriched services provided at CCRCs, it is not surprising that the cost of living for CCRC residents in ILUs (apartments, cottages, or town houses) appeared to be a little higher for persons with a higher-level budget in the general community.

distinguish extended from limited CCRCs will affect decisions regarding CCRC entrance.

Organizationally, for example, limited CCRCs incur less financial risk than extended CCRCs for providing nursing home care to their residents. The closer the arrangement is to a fee-for-service plan, the more feasible it becomes for limited facilities to accept vulnerable individuals as apartment dwellers — that is, persons with functional impairments or medical problems that put them at risk for institutional placement within the foreseeable future.

Along with less financial risk when members of the population need to be transferred permanently to the health center (nursing home), the organizational data also indicated that fewer supportive services were included in the monthly fees of limited CCRCs. In general, more supportive services that might be needed or desired by residents were paid for by the resident strictly on a fee-for-service basis. This might account in part for the generally lower monthly fees charged by limited CCRCs.

Differences in costs to potential residents can be expected to affect choice. Thus, regardless of the attractiveness of the pooled-risk philosophy to individuals interested in the CCRC living arrangement, higher entrance and particularly higher ongoing monthly fees for their apartments may have limited the population for whom extended CCRCs could be considered an economically feasible option.

Even aside from an individual's financial status, in line with philosophical differences regarding pooled risk as an insurance against potential costly nursing home placement, to some persons the provision of meals, housecleaning, laundry, and transportation may have made extended CCRCs seem particularly attractive. These supportive services may have been considered amenities or preventive measures rather than strictly services needed because of functional impairments.

Alternatively, CCRCs providing care on a fee-for-service basis may meet the needs of those who desire to select from a menu of services. On an ongoing basis, more of the residents of limited CCRCs may prefer to pay only for supportive services that they themselves desire and use. These persons would also be more willing to risk the possibility of future expenses for nursing home care rather than pay for the insurance provided by pooled risk. Also, somewhat mitigating the anticipation of potential huge increases in health care costs, the residents of the limited CCRCs were more likely to have an intermediate living arrangement option (personal care or assisted living unit) available to them when they no longer were able to manage in their own apartments but did not need the more expensive higher-level services provided by a nursing home.

Extended and limited CCRCs were generally similar in terms of commitment to their residents in the case of an unexpected reversal of financial status. Of the structural features examined, religious affiliation, availability of nursing home beds (as measured by the proportion of beds to apartments), and Medicare/Medicaid certification did not seem to differentiate between the two types of facility. It was not expected, therefore, that these features would be related to distinctions that might be found between the personal characteristics of those who chose either type of CCRC.

The size of the community, however, was a characteristic that distinguished between extended and limited CCRCs. Compared with only three of the extended CCRCs, seven of the ten limited CCRCs had considerably fewer than 250 apartments (two of which were under 200 apartments). Compared with only one limited CCRC, six of the extended CCRCs had more than 300 apartments (two of which had more than 500 apartments). Persons selecting the limited CCRCs may have been looking for a small- to moderate-size community; in other words, persons selecting the extended rather than the limited CCRCs may have been more willing to enter large communities.

The limited CCRCs were also distinguished from the extended CCRCs in this study by the fact that one of its numbers had been in existence for 96 years in 1986. This was a 100 percent occupied CCRC organized on an almost complete fee-for-service basis, including both supportive services to apartment dwellers and long-term care in their nursing home. Although it had a mid-range entrance fee, it had the lowest monthly fee ($296 in 1986), and its nursing home beds were Medicaid as well as Medicare certified, making the facility particularly attractive to persons with limited annual incomes.

The occupancy rate was on average lower for limited CCRCs but tended nevertheless to be relatively high. In one of the two limited CCRCs with lower than than 80 percent occupancy, the vacant units were primarily studio apartments; this CCRC was in the process of converting these apartments into assisted living (personal care) units. The low rate in the second CCRC may also have reflected a temporary situation. Although remaining a nonprofit CCRC, the second CCRC was experiencing a change in sponsorship and management. It is possible that the occupancy rate of this CCRC will rise if a positive reputation of the sponsor and manager becomes established. Until the occupancy rate increases in these two CCRCs, it does not seem likely that they will take financial risk by relaxing criteria regarding financial solvency of applicants in order to fill vacant apartments. Since limited CCRCs are generally at lower financial risk for nursing home care, they also might not need as high a rate of occupancy to remain solvent.

Comparison of the Residents of the Two Types of CCRC
Study Samples, Data Sources, and Analyses

The samples for these analyses consisted of the recent and longer-stay residents in the randomly drawn study samples who met two criteria. First, residents were living in apartments or other ILUs of the CCRC at baseline. Second, they had both baseline and follow-up interviews approximately sixteen months later. The samples included residents under 70 as well as those 70 years of age or older. The study sample of recent residents consisted of 281 drawn from extended CCRCs and 220 from limited CCRCs; the study sample of longer-stay residents consisted of 549 individuals from extended CCRCs and 579 from limited CCRCs.

We gathered both entrance and baseline information on characteristics from the in-depth baseline resident interviews. Directly pertinent to understanding similarities and differences between residents choosing these different types of CCRC are the analyses of available data about characteristics at the time of and before entrance. The entrance characteristics data set included thirteen items: how the respondents learned about the CCRC (from informal or other sources); whether the residents had visited other CCRCs before choosing the CCRC in which they resided; and eleven demographic characteristics covering age and sex of the residents, religious affiliation, place of birth, educational status, whether the residents lived alone on entrance to the CCRC; four aspects of their residence before entering the CCRC; and whether or not they were in the work force for most of their lives.

The data set used to compare resident characteristics at the first interview consisted of twenty-four variables. Ten of these were demographic characteristics and variables related to informal support: age at baseline; whether living alone at baseline; four marital status variables (the percentages in each category were analyzed separately) — whether still married, widowed, divorced/separated, or never married; number of children; residential distance (propinquity) of children and of other relatives; and number of informal helpers (either currently providing or could be counted on to provide help if needed). Four variables were relevant to financing the CCRC living arrangement, and two were relevant to other expenditures (medical and outside entertainment). Eight were measures of health and functional status, including the number of medical problems; two questions were about perceived health, whether the resident had ever had a nursing home stay; and four were summary scales regarding medical problems, impairments in personal activities of daily living (ADL), instrumental activities of daily living (IADL), mobility, and a self-sufficiency index.

We asked sample members twenty-two questions about their reasons for entering the CCRC, eight questions at baseline and the remainder during follow-up. In addition to the individual items, we developed reasons-for-entrance scales through factor analysis and standardized alpha reliability techniques. Later we will describe the scoring for the eight baseline and fourteen follow-up questions, the methods used to develop the scales, and their scoring systems.

In the statistical analyses of entrance and baseline characteristics and reasons for entrance, we compared the samples of residents of extended CCRCs with those who lived in limited CCRCs. To determine the significance of the difference between groups of residents we used chi-square analysis to examine differences in percentages and analyses of variance (ANOVAs) to determine the significance of mean differences. In one set of analyses, we compared living arrangement (whether living alone or not) at entrance with living arrangement at baseline; significance level calculations in these comparisons were based on McNemar's Z for correlated proportions. As we said in Chapter 1, we considered differences at the $p \leq 0.05$ level significant.

Comparisons between Residents of Extended and Limited CCRCs at Entrance

Table 2.1 describes and compares the baseline characteristics of recent and longer-stay residents by type of CCRC. In general, the response patterns were similar for recent and longer-stay residents in the two types of CCRC. For example, if a large proportion of recent residents in extended CCRCs had a particular characteristic, a large proportion of longer-stay residents usually had that characteristic too. Nevertheless, there were some statistically significant differences in entrance characteristics between residents of extended and limited CCRCs — fewer for the recent residents than for the longer-stay residents of the two types of CCRC.

Consistent Nonsignificant Differences. There were no significant differences between recent residents of extended and limited CCRCs or between longer-stay residents in these two types of facility in five of the thirteen entrance characteristics. Namely, sizable proportions in each sample (more than 43 percent of the recent and more than half of the longer-stay residents) lived alone at admission. Even larger proportions — well over half of each sample — were female (at least 68 percent of the recent and 78 percent of the longer-stay residents), had participated in the work force (84 to 85 percent), had visited other CCRCs before select-

Table 2.1 Entrance characteristics of residents, by CCRC type

	Recent (< one year)		Longer-stay	
	Extended (N = 281)	Limited (N = 220)	Extended[a] (N = 549)	Limited[b] (N = 579)
Learned about CCRC from informal sources (%)[c]	72.6	77.7	71.8*	66.1
Visited other CCRCs before selecting one (%)	58.4	64.1	59.0	62.0
Mean age at admission	77.9	78.4	76.3*	77.1
Female (%)	67.6	69.5	78.3	78.4
Protestant (%)	82.6	85.9	86.7*	94.1
Foreign born (%)	3.2*	7.3	5.8	7.9
College graduate (%)[d]	54.8*	38.6	61.4*	47.5
Mean years of education	15.2*	13.7	15.2*	14.5
Lived alone at admission (%)	43.1	46.8	50.5	53.5
Prior residence (at entrance)				
Private house (%)	49.8*	57.7	49.0*	53.5
Retirement community (%)[e]	17.8*	10.5	22.6*	12.6
Owned own home before CCRC entrance (%)	70.8	76.8	69.9	73.9
In work force during adult years (%)	84.3	84.5	84.9	84.4

Note. Analyzed separately for recent and longer-stay residents. An asterisk following the column for residents in extended CCRCs indicates that the difference between residents in extended and limited CCRCs was statistically significant at the < 0.05 level.

[a]Significant differences between recent and longer-stay residents of extended CCRCs were found for age at admission, being female, and living alone at admission.

[b]Significant differences between recent and longer-stay residents of limited CCRCs were found for whether they learned about the CCRC from informal sources, age at admission, years of education, being female, college graduate, and living alone at admission.

[c]Informal sources included friends, neighbors, relatives, and church referrals. Other-than-informal sources included newspapers, magazines, unsolicited announcements, TV or radio, and other.

[d]The college graduate category included persons with more than a college education along with those with a college education.

[e]Included another CCRC or other retirement community.

ing the facility in which they currently lived (more than 58 percent), and had owned their own home (70 percent or more).

We should note that although sex distribution and the percent of residents who lived alone at entrance did not distinguish between recent and longer-stay residents of extended and limited CCRCs, there were consistent differences in these characteristics between recent and longer-stay residents within each type of facility. For both extended and limited CCRCs more of the longer-stay residents were female, and more lived alone at entrance.

Consistent Differences. There were two differences in prior residence in the samples from extended and limited CCRCs. Regardless of whether or not the residents owned their homes, significantly larger proportions of those who entered limited CCRCs came from a private house in an age-integrated community (57 and 54 percent, respectively, of the recent and longer-stay residents in limited CCRCs compared with 50 percent of the recent and 49 percent of the longer-stay residents in extended CCRCs). Conversely, although only a minority in each of the groups moved to the CCRC from another retirement community, proportionately more of those moving to extended CCRCs had done so[4] (18 percent of the recent and 23 percent of the longer-stay residents of extended CCRCs and 11 and 18 percent of the recent and longer-stay residents of limited CCRCs). It appears that more individuals moving into extended CCRCs had prior experience living in an age-segregated (older adult) community.

There were also consistent educational differences between residents in the two types of CCRC. Notwithstanding a relatively high level of education in all sample groups, both in terms of the percent with a college degree and the mean number of years of education, residents of extended CCRCs tended to be better educated than those of limited facilities. In limited CCRCs the educational status of the recent residents was significantly lower than that of the longer-stay residents.

Mixed Findings. For three variables there were differences between longer-stay but not recent residents in the two types of community. These included age at entrance, religion, and whether the resident had learned about the CCRC from informal sources. The statistically significant dif-

4. Very few came from other CCRCs. Only 7 of the total sample of 501 recent entrants came from other CCRCs, 5 of the 281 residents from extended CCRCs, and 2 of the 220 residents from limited CCRCs. Seven of the total sample of 1,128 longer-stay residents had entered from another CCRC, 3 of the 549 residents from extended CCRCs, and 4 of the 579 residents from limited CCRCs.

ference in mean age at entrance between the two groups of longer-stay residents was about nine and a half months — a mean age of 76.3 years for residents of extended CCRCs and 77.1 years for residents of limited CCRCs. Although the difference was not statistically significant, the recent residents of extended CCRCs were younger at admission (by about six months) than their limited CCRC counterparts (77.9 and 78.4 years of age at admission, respectively). In one respect, age at entrance followed a consistent pattern in both types of CCRC: the recent residents were on average more than a year older at admission than were the longer-stay residents, and in each case the difference was statistically significant.

Less than 18 percent in any of the samples were non-Protestant. Among the longer-stay residents, however, there was more than twice the proportion of non-Protestants in extended than in limited CCRCs — 13 percent compared with 6 percent. In fact, the proportion of Protestants among recent residents of limited CCRCs (86 percent) was significantly lower than among longer-stay residents of these facilities (94 percent) and more similar to both the recent (83 percent) and longer-stay residents (87 percent) of extended CCRCs.

In addition, a majority in each sample had learned about the facility from informal/personal sources such as friends, relatives, and church referrals rather than from the media or other sources, including newspapers, television, radio, and unsolicited announcements. Nevertheless, except for place of birth, for each of these characteristics there were significant differences between longer-stay residents in the two types of CCRC but *not* between recent residents. Significantly more longer-stay residents of extended rather than limited CCRCs (72 and 66 percent, respectively) learned about the community from friends, neighbors, relatives, or their church. In contrast to the other entrance variables, not only was the difference between recent residents not statistically significant, but the pattern of the difference between the groups was not similar. Even more of the recent limited (78 percent) than extended (73 percent) CCRC residents had learned about the facility from informal sources; at least 10 percent more of the recent than longer-stay residents of limited CCRCs had learned about the facility from these sources, and this difference was statistically significant.

For one variable, place of birth, there was a statistically significant difference between samples, but in this case, only between recent residents in the two types of CCRC. Although the percentages were very small, a slightly higher percentage of the recent residents of limited CCRCs was foreign born — 7 percent compared with 3 percent of the recent residents of extended CCRCs.

Comparisons between Residents of Extended and
Limited CCRCs at Baseline

We gathered comparable data about entrance and baseline characteristics only for age and living arrangement (whether lived alone). Since the baseline occurred some time after entrance, the mean age of the sample members would have changed by baseline, particularly the average age of the longer-stay residents. On average, at baseline recent residents of extended and limited CCRCs were approximately 4.3 and 6 months older, respectively, than they were at admission; for longer-stay residents, the difference between admission and baseline age was 5 years 7.4 months for extended and 5 years 10.3 months for limited CCRC residents. Living arrangements changed very little for recent residents. But a statistically significant proportion — 12 and 13 percent, respectively, of the extended and limited CCRCs longer-stay sample members — changed their living situation between admission and baseline (having a partner at admission but living alone at baseline). Therefore, for the recent residents the baseline information could be assumed to have provided a reasonably accurate estimate of the individual's status at entrance. But this was not so for the longer-stay residents.

Table 2.2 describes and compares the baseline characteristics of recent and longer-stay residents by type of CCRC. In the separate comparisons made between recent residents of extended and limited CCRCs and between longer-stay residents in the two types of community, there were no significant differences, in either type of facility, for one third of the baseline characteristics examined. However, there were differences between residents of extended and limited CCRCs for almost one third. In one instance, there was a difference between recent but not longer-stay residents, and there were differences between longer-stay residents in the two types of CCRC but not between recent residents for the remaining third of these background characteristics.

Consistent Similarities. Of the eight background characteristics in this category, there were no significant differences in six demographic characteristics between residents in the two types of CCRC. These characteristics included whether the resident lived alone at baseline, three of the four marital status categories (the percentages married, separated or divorced, and never married), and the two residential propinquity variables (mean number of children within a one-hour drive and the mean number of relatives within a one-hour drive).

Fifty percent or more of the recent residents were still married and

Table 2.2 Baseline characteristics of residents, by CCRC type

	Recent (< one year)		Longer-stay	
	Extended (N = 281)	Limited (N = 220)	Extended[a] (N = 549)	Limited[b] (N = 579)
Baseline mean years of age	78.2	78.9	82.0*	82.9
Lived alone at baseline (%)	43.8	50.5	60.8	65.3
Mean no. of live children	1.39	1.30	1.05*	1.24
Marital status[c]				
Married (%)	54.4	49.8	37.5	33.9
Widowed (%)	33.5*	42.3	45.5*	51.5
Separated/divorced (%)	3.9	0.8	1.8	2.8
Never married (%)	8.2	6.8	15.1	11.9
Residential propinquity of relatives				
Mean no. of children within a 1-hour drive	0.49	0.45	0.30	0.34
Mean no. of relatives within a 1-hour drive	3.63	3.16	2.26	1.89
No. of informal helpers or potential helpers (up to 4)	2.82	2.88	2.24*	2.43
Relevant to financing CCRC living arrangement				
Annual income over $30,000[d] (%)	52.3	48.2	52.8*	38.7
Income from investments (%)	98.6*	95.0	97.1*	93.4
Draws upon to finance monthly fee				
Interest (from savings, investments, trust funds) (%)	67.6*	45.5	61.4*	54.7
Principal (savings, trust funds, proceeds from sale of property) (%)	8.5*	1.8	4.7	2.9

Table 2.2 Continued

Other expenditures				
Out-of-pocket medical expenses last month (%)				
(0) None	22.8	10.9	16.4	13.8
(1) Less than $100	59.8*	68.2	71.2*	64.8
(2) $100+	17.4	20.9	12.4	21.4
Regularly spends money on outside entertainment	62.3*	39.5	54.9*	35.9
Health and functional status				
Mean no. of medical problems[e] (0–10)	2.08*	2.37	2.30*	2.59
Health rating [(1) Excellent . . . (4) Poor]	1.81*	2.03	1.95*	2.03
Change in health (%)				
(1) Worse than a year ago	8.6	15.0	12.6	16.5
(2) Same	83.6	77.3	83.4	77.8
(3) Better	7.9	7.7	4.0	5.7
Had never been a nursing home patient (%)	95.0	94.5	88.9*	77.7
Mean ADL impairment scale[f] (0–5)	0.26	0.29	0.33*	0.51*
Mobility impairment index[g] (0–6)	0.18	0.21	0.34*	0.51
Mean IADL index[h] (0–6)	0.85	0.88	1.10	1.19
Mean self-sufficiency score[i] (1–4)	1.29	1.25	1.34*	1.49

Note. Analyzed separately for recent and longer-stay residents, an asterisk following the column for residents in extended CCRCs indicates that the difference between residents in extended and limited CCRCs was statistically significant at the ≤ 0.05 level.

[a]Significant differences were found between recent and longer-stay residents of extended CCRCs for all but separated/divorced, income over $30,000, and income from investments, and scores of the ADL impairment and self-sufficiency scales.

[b]Significant differences were found between recent and longer-stay residents of extended CCRCs for all but no. of live children, separated/divorced, income from investments, drawing upon principal to finance monthly fee, out-of-pocket medical expenses, regularly spends money on outside entertainment, and the three health and financial status variables.

[c]The chi-squares for marital status when all four categories were included in the calculations yield p levels of 0.147 for the comparison between recent residents of extended and limited CCRCs and 0.095 for the comparison of longer-stay residents.

[d]The same pattern and significance of difference between the two CCRC type longer-stay residents were found for percent over $20,000. Categories for income were: <$20,000, $20,001 to $30,000, $30,001 to $40,000, $40,001 to $50,000, and over $50,000.

[e]A count of the following ten medical problems: arthritis, high blood pressure, heart problem, diabetes, stroke, neurological conditions (other than Alzheimer's or related dementias, e.g., Parkinson's, palsies), cancer, orthopedic conditions, emphysema or other lung (pulmonary) condition, and circulatory or vascular problems (blood clots, varicose veins, phlebitis, etc.).

[f]ADL impairment index: from 0 (no impairments) to 5 (most impairments), no of problems in the following: dressing, bathing, personal care, transfer out of a chair, and managing medications.

[g]Mobility impairment scale score 0 to 6 problem areas (high score, more problems): uses walker/wheelchair, problem in climbing stairs, wheeling twenty feet; wheeling a half-mile, walking twenty feet, walking a half-mile (wheeling not considered a problem area if walks a half-mile).

[h]IADL index: scored from 0 to 6 (higher score, more problems), indicating the respondent needed some help most or all of the time regarding (most importantly) meal preparation, ordinary work around the house such as light housekeeping, shopping and tasks such as taking out garbage and small errands, and (less importantly) heavy housecleaning and similar chores.

[i]Self-sufficiency index scored from 1 to 4: 1, self-sufficient . . . 4, least self-sufficient. Score 1, can have up to one IADL, ADL, or mobility problem, but it does not prevent the individual from going out of the house two or more days a week, nor does bad health, sickness, or pain prevent the individual from performing desired activities. Score 2, either has two such problems or has only one such problem but also has a problem going out of house or is prevented by health, sickness, or pain from performing desired activities. Score 3, in addition to having one or the other minimal conditions that would be scored as 2, would have an additional IADL, ADL, or mobility problem. Score 4, having more problems than described above.

did not live alone at baseline. Very few were divorced/separated (less than 4 percent in any of the groups) or never married (7 to 8 percent for the recent residents and 12 to 15 percent for the longer-stay residents). Many persons had no children living within a one-hour drive of their community. The average number of children nearby was considerably lower than one in each of the groups (an average of 0.49 and 0.45 children, respectively, for recent residents of extended and limited CCRCs, and 0.30 and 0.34 for the longer-stay residents). Not including children or spouses, residents did tend to have other relatives nearby — an average of 3.63 and 3.16 relatives within a one-hour drive for recent residents of extended and limited CCRCs, respectively, and 2.26 and 1.89 relatives for the longer-stay residents.

In addition to these six variables, there were no significant differences between residents of extended and limited CCRCs, either recent or longer-stay residents, for two health and functional status variables: perceived change in health and problems in instrumental activities of daily living as measured by the IADL impairment index. More than three quarters in each of the two CCRC groups reported no change in health over the past year. Although some in each group reported a change for the better, more noted a change for the worse. In general, both recent and longer-stay residents exhibited few impairments in IADL (scores range from 0 to 6 on the IADL impairment index with 0 denoting no problems). On average, recent residents scored lower than 1, and longer-stay residents, only a little over 1.

Consistent Differences. There were significant differences between extended and limited CCRC residents in two health variables: number of medical problems and self-perceived rating of health. The mean number of medical problems (of ten) was considerably lower than 2.5 in all but the longer-stay limited CCRC sample. Yet differences between recent residents of extended and limited CCRCs were significant as well as the differences between the longer-stay residents in the two types of CCRC. In each instance, on average, residents of extended CCRCs had fewer medical problems than did those of limited facilities (a mean of 2.08 and 2.37, respectively, for recent residents of extended and limited CCRCs, and 2.30 and 2.59 medical problems, respectively, for the longer-stay residents). Similarly, although the mean self-rated health of residents of limited type was relatively high (in the "good" range) in all sample groups, in the comparison between recent residents and between longer-stay residents of the two types of CCRC, extended CCRC residents tended to report better health than their counterparts in limited CCRCs.

Widowhood was the only marital status variable for which there was a difference between residents of extended and limited CCRC residents. More than one third in all of the samples were widowed (closer to half among the longer-stay residents), but in each of the comparisons, significantly fewer residents of extended CCRCs than of limited CCRCs were widowed.

There were consistent differences between extended and limited CCRC residents in two characteristics relevant to financing the CCRC living arrangement. Although a very large majority (more than 93 percent) in each sample group had income from investments, in each comparison this was the case for a higher percentage of the extended CCRC residents. In line with these findings, a higher percentage of extended CCRC residents drew upon interest from savings, investments, or trust funds to finance the monthly fee: of the recent residents, 68 percent of the extended and 46 percent of the limited CCRC residents; of the longer-stay residents, 61 and 55 percent, respectively.

The final two characteristics for which there were consistent differences between residents of the two types of CCRC focused on out-of-pocket expenditures: medical expenses above and beyond what was received from Medicare and/or health insurance; and, aside from vacations, whether the resident spent money regularly for entertainment outside the home, for example, for movies, plays, concerts, and sporting events.

In the month before baseline, the majority of residents in each of the groups spent less than $100 on medical expenses. Yet residents of limited CCRCs tended to have significantly more out-of-pocket medical expenses than did the residents of extended CCRCs in that month. Among recent residents, greater than twice the proportion of extended (23 percent) than limited CCRC residents (11 percent) had *no* out-of-pocket medical expenses. Among longer-stay residents, as many as 21 percent of those in limited CCRCs had $100 or more of out-of-pocket medical expenses compared with 12 percent of the residents of extended CCRCs. It is possible that the greater amount of out-of-pocket money spent by residents of limited CCRCs may have been the result of poorer health.

In contrast, proportionately more of the residents in the extended than limited communities spent money regularly on outside entertainment — 62 and 40 percent, respectively, of the recent residents, and 55 and 36 percent of the longer-stay residents of extended and limited CCRCs. Since there was little difference in the amenities provided by the extended and limited CCRCs studied, the larger proportion of both recent and longer-stay residents of extended CCRCs who spent money regularly on outside entertainment may have reflected differences in life style and/or economic status.

Differences between Longer-Stay but Not between Recent Residents. There were fewer statistically significant differences between the samples of recent residents in the extended and limited CCRCs than between the samples of longer-stay residents. However, with one exception — the number of living children — the pattern of differences between recent residents of extended and limited CCRCs was similar to that found in the comparisons of longer-stay residents. On average, longer-stay residents of limited CCRCs had a significantly greater number of living children (1.24) than did longer-stay residents of extended CCRCs (1.08). In addition, the number of living children of recent residents of extended CCRCs was a little larger (1.39) than that found for recent residents of limited CCRCs (1.30).

The following describes the differences between residents of extended and limited CCRCs which were significant only in the comparison of longer-stay residents but which followed a similar pattern between recent residents in the two types of CCRC:

- Longer-stay residents in extended CCRCs tended to be slightly younger (an average age of 82 years) than those in limited CCRCs (82.9 years).
- Longer-stay extended CCRC residents tended to have fewer informal helpers (or potential helpers) who could be counted on (a mean of 2.24 helpers) than their counterparts in limited CCRCs (2.43 helpers).
- A large majority of recent and longer-stay residents in both types of CCRC had never been a nursing home patient, but more of the longer-stay residents of extended than of limited CCRCs had never been a nursing home patient (89 percent compared with 78 percent for the residents of limited CCRCs).
- Although few residents in any of the groups had ADL impairments, the longer-stay residents of extended CCRCs also had fewer ADL impairments (on average, 0.33 impairments) than did the longer-stay residents of limited CCRCs (0.51 impairments).
- Extended residents had better scores on the self-sufficiency scale than did those in limited CCRCs (with lower scores indicative of greater self-sufficiency, a mean of 1.34 for longer-stay extended CCRC residents compared with 1.49 in limited CCRCs).
- Although the majority in all of the samples (recent and longer-stay) had little or no mobility problems, the longer-stay extended CCRC residents tended to have fewer of them than their counterparts in limited CCRCs. Of six mobility problems in the index, the extended

CCRC residents had a mean of 0.34 and the limited CCRC residents a mean of 0.51.

▪ A higher percentage of longer-stay residents in extended (53 percent) than in limited CCRCs (39 percent) had incomes of more than $30,000 at baseline.

Difference between Recent but Not between Longer-Stay Residents. The one variable for which there was a significant difference between recent but not between the longer-stay residents of the two types of CCRC was whether or not the resident used the principal from savings or trust funds or the proceeds from the sale of property to finance the CCRC monthly fee. Although very few in any of the groups (recent or longer-stay) used principal to finance the monthly fee, more of the recent residents of extended CCRCs (9 percent) than of limited CCRCs (2 percent) did so.

Reasons for Entering a CCRC

The reasons that residents gave for having chosen their CCRC may point to similarities and differences between persons who selected an extended rather than a limited CCRC. As in the comparisons of residents at entrance and at baseline, we will present data regarding both recent and longer-stay residents. There were significant differences between residents of extended and limited CCRCs as well as between recent and longer-stay residents within each type of CCRC. Note that within-CCRC differences do not necessarily signify that reasons for entrance are changing. Clearly, the greater the distance in time between entrance and baseline, the greater the chance that experience and memory factors might have entered into retrospectively claimed reasons for entrance. Thus, an alternate and equally plausible hypothesis to explain differences between recent and longer-stay residents within either CCRC type is that perceptions regarding motivation for moving to the CCRC may have changed over time. From this perspective, the separate comparisons of recent residents and longer-stay residents by CCRC type are more meaningful, and the responses of recent residents regarding why they chose the CCRC are particularly interesting.

Measures of Reasons for Entrance

We asked sample members a series of twenty-two questions regarding their reasons for entering the CCRC: eight questions at baseline and fourteen at follow-up, approximately sixteen months after baseline. The baseline interview included reasons for their decision to live in the CCRC they chose (calling for a *yes* or *no* response). The follow-up questions included whether each of fourteen reasons was important (*very, somewhat,* or *not important*) in the decision. These reasons were more specific about some of the baseline areas and included additional dimensions as well. Although the questions were asked somewhat differently at baseline and at follow-up, all attempted to get at the issue of why the residents chose the CCRC in which they currently resided.

The baseline interview included the following eight reasons for living in a particular CCRC: desirability of apartment/location; wanting to live with people similar to oneself; access to needed services — now and in the future; proximity to friends/relatives or a familiar area; protective features guaranteed in the contract; compensation for the absence or potential absence of helpers; avoidance of pressure/demands on family or friends; and a guarantee of living within one's means (asset protection). The percent of residents who indicated that a particular reason applied to them are shown below. Based on the chi-square statistic, there were differences that were significant at the $p \leq 0.05$ level between residents of extended and limited CCRCs as well as between recent and longer-stay residents within each type of CCRC.

During the follow-up interview we asked the residents about the importance of the following fourteen reasons in choosing their CCRC: a nice apartment unit; extensive common areas; high-quality image and decor; location; security and safety; housekeeping services available; meals available in the dining room; personal care services available; nursing home available; maintenance and yard work done; system for handling medical emergencies; transportation furnished; fees included nursing home care; and guaranteed residence even if income drops.

In presenting the data regarding the questions asked at follow-up, we combined the responses *very* and *somewhat important* so that the frame of reference was more like that of the baseline questions. However, we conducted similar analyses in which we compared the similarities and differences between samples in the proportions who considered each of these fourteen reasons to be very important. We will present findings from both of these comparisons, noting significant differences when they occur.

We also used these items to develop reasons-for-entrance scales. As a first step in doing so, we factor analyzed the reasons probed at baseline and at follow-up using the combined samples of recent and longer-stay residents ($N = 1,629$). For each of the factors identified, we defined as a set those questions with factor loadings greater than 0.4. We then constructed scales (indices) by adding response scores and testing for alpha reliability; we considered unacceptable a standardized alpha reliability of 0.5 or lower.

Since the scales contained different numbers of questions, we computed another score. For each of the scales, referred to as *proportions scales*, we divided the summed score by the maximum score possible for that scale. We drew conclusions regarding the importance of each of the scale domains based on the ordering of these scales.

Baseline Reasons for Entrance

Table 2.3 compares residents in extended and limited CCRCs as to the eight reasons for entrance which were asked in the baseline interview. Although residents responded inconsistently regarding desirable apartment/location and wanting to be with people like themselves, more than half of the recent and longer-stay resident samples from both types of CCRC claimed that each of the remaining six reasons probed at baseline applied to them. Nevertheless, for most of these variables there were significant differences between the recent residents of extended and limited CCRCs, between the longer-stay residents, or both.

Among recent residents, access to needed services ranked very high as a reason for entrance, regardless of CCRC type. It was the most pervasive of the eight reasons applying to their decision to live in the CCRC that they had chosen; 92 percent of recent residents in extended and 87 percent of those in limited CCRCs said this reason applied to them, and the difference between these samples was not statistically significant. Guaranteed protective features of the contract also ranked very high among recent residents of both types of CCRC (the second most pervasive reason), although in this case significantly more of the recent residents of extended CCRCs (88 percent) than of limited CCRCs (78 percent) said that this reason applied to their choice of living arrangement.

Both of these reasons also ranked high among longer-stay residents, with generally more than three quarters in these samples saying that these reasons influenced their decision to enter the CCRC. There were significant differences, however, between longer-stay residents of extended and limited CCRCs for each of these reasons. A higher percent of those in limited (85 percent) than in extended CCRCs (78 percent) said that access to needed services entered into their decision, but a higher percent of the longer-stay extended CCRC residents (87 percent compared with 73 percent of the limited CCRC residents) said that guaranteed protective features of the contract influenced their decision. It is not clear why fewer of the longer-stay residents of extended than of limited

Table 2.3 Reasons for entrance (queried at baseline)

	Recent		Longer-stay	
	Extended (N = 281)	Limited (N = 220)	Extended[a] (N = 549)	Limited[b] (N = 579)
	%	%	%	%
Desirable apartment/location	58.4*	69.5	48.3**	69.8
Desire to be with people like myself	38.8*	52.3	43.1**	53.7
Access to needed services now and in future	91.5	87.3	77.5**	85.1
To live close to friends/relatives or near familiar area	54.8**	72.3	50.5*	59.8
Guranteed protective features of contract	87.5*	77.7	87.1**	73.1
Compensation for absence or potential absence of helper	53.4*	65.5	54.1**	63.6
Avoid pressure/demands on family or friends	77.9	73.2	63.4	62.3
To guarantee living within means (to protect assets/to be independent)	71.5	70.0	65.0**	75.0

Note. Analyzed separately for recent and longer-stay residents, an asterisk following the column for residents in extended CCRCs indicates that the difference between residents in extended and limited CCRCs was statistically significant at $p \leq 0.01$. Two asterisks following the column for residents in extended CCRCs indicates that the difference between residents in extended and limited CCRCs was statistically significant at $p \leq 0.001$.

[a]Significant differences were found between recent and longer-stay residents of extended CCRCs for the following reasons: desirable apartment, access to needed services, and to avoid personal demands on family or friends.

[b]Significant differences were found between recent and longer-stay residents of limited CCRCs for the following reasons: to live close to friends/relatives and to avoid personal demands on family or friends.

CCRCs claimed access to needed services as a reason for entrance since this was a feature of both types of contract; in fact, this pattern of difference was reversed among recent residents in the two types of CCRC. However, the significantly higher percent of residents of extended CCRCs (both recent and longer-stay) than of limited CCRCs reporting that guaranteed protective features of the contract influenced them certainly makes sense since this is a much stronger feature of the extended than of the limited CCRC contract.

Large, but not significantly different, percentages of the recent residents of the extended and limited CCRC residents (78 and 73 percent, respectively) said that one of the reasons for entrance was to avoid pressure and demands on family or friends. Although proportionately fewer than among the recent residents, a majority of the longer-stay residents in the two types of CCRC also made this claim (63 percent of the extended and 62 percent of the limited CCRC residents), and the difference was not significant.

A large and similar proportion of the recent residents in the two types of CCRC—as many as 72 percent of the recent residents of extended CCRCs and 70 percent of the residents of limited CCRCs—gave the guarantee of living within one's means (to protect assets and to be independent) as a reason for entering the CCRC. Among longer-stay residents, however, there was a significant difference: only 65 percent of extended CCRC residents compared with 75 percent of the residents of limited CCRCs gave this as a reason for their choice.

Significantly more of the residents of limited than of extended CCRCs, regardless of length of stay, also said that the following were among their reasons for choosing this type of living arrangement: living close to friends/relatives or near a familiar area; desirable apartment/location; to compensate for the absence or potential absence of helpers; and their desire to be with people like themselves.

In all groups, the desire to be with people like themselves ranked lowest among the eight reasons. Significantly fewer in extended than in limited CCRCs indicated this as a consideration in their choosing the CCRC—38.8 percent of recent and 43.1 percent of longer-stay residents of extended CCRCs, in contrast with as many as 52.3 percent of recent and 53.7 percent of longer-stay residents of limited CCRCs.[5]

Follow-up Reasons for Entrance

The residents' responses in the follow-up interview (approximately sixteen months after baseline) provided further insights into similarities and differences in their reasons for selecting the extended or limited CCRCs. Table 2.4 compares these responses. By this time, of course, recent residents had been in the CCRC for longer than a year, and longer-

---

5. There were several within-CCRC type differences between recent and longer-stay residents. Significantly more of the recent than the longer-stay residents in both types of CCRCs said that avoiding pressure on their family or friends was a reason for entrance. More of the recent than of the longer-stay residents of limited CCRCs said that proximity to friends or relatives was a reason. More of the recent than of the longer-stay residents of extended CCRCs said that a desirable apartment location and access to needed services entered into their decision to join the community.

Table 2.4 Reasons considered important (very important) in CCRC choice (queried at follow-up)

	Recent		Longer-stay	
	Extended (N = 281)	Limited (N = 220)	Extended[a] (N = 549)	Limited[b] (N = 579)
	%	%	%	%
A nice apartment unit				
Important	91.1	85.9	89.4	87.9
Very important	71.9	74.3	68.0	72.7
Extensive common areas				
Important	76.5	72.3	75.4	71.8
Very important	34.5*	43.3	37.8	39.4
High-quality image/decor				
Important	86.1*	78.6	86.5	82.6
Very important	48.8	56.1	54.6	52.2
Location				
Important	81.9	85.5	82.3	86.2
Very important	65.8	69.8	68.1	71.4
Availability of housekeeping services				
Important	85.1*	66.8	86.0*	67.2
Very important	55.4*	36.3	56.4*	43.0
Meals in dining room				
Important	88.6*	65.9	88.7*	72.2
Very important	66.1*	46.0	63.3*	53.7
Personal care services				
Important	87.5*	80.0	89.3*	73.2
Very important	80.4*	66.4	80.9*	58.1
Nursing home				
Important	94.3*	84.5	95.3*	78.1
Very important	88.6*	73.0	92.1*	70.6
Maintenance and yard work done				
Important	81.1	75.9	84.7*	77.0
Very important	63.7*	54.0	61.3	60.5
Security/safety				
Important	81.1*	62.3	75.0*	67.5
Very important	59.4*	47.2	56.3	54.1
System for handling medical emergencies				
Important	96.1*	89.5	93.1*	86.7
Very important	91.1	86.0	89.1*	80.6

Table 2.4 Continued

	Recent		Longer-stay	
	Extended (N = 281)	Limited (N = 220)	Extended[a] (N = 549)	Limited[b] (N = 579)
	%	%	%	%
Transportation furnished				
Important	54.1	49.1	59.4*	45.3
Very important	38.1	30.4	48.0*	29.7*
Fees include nursing home care				
Important	90.0*	32.3	89.8*	36.1
Very important	84.0*	21.6	84.8*	25.7
Guaranteed residence even if income drops				
Important	75.1*	46.8	73.8*	52.7
Very important	66.9*	40.2	62.6*	42.2

Note. For comparisons between residents of extended and limited CCRCs, separately for recent and longer-stay residents, an asterisk to the right of the column depicting the percentage of residents of extended CCRCs indicates that the difference between the two groups was statistically significant at the ≤ 0.05 probability level.

[a]Significant differences were found between recent and longer-stay residents of extended CCRCs in persons saying that security/safety and transportation furnished were important.

[b]Significant differences were found between recent and longer-stay residents of limited CCRCS in the percentage saying that personal care services were important and very important and in the percentage saying that the availability of a nursing home was important.

stay residents, for at least two years. Although it was advisable to consider the baseline and follow-up responses separately because of the difference in the point in time when these questions were asked, the generally parallel pattern of similarities and differences between residents of extended and limited CCRCs, regardless of length of stay, suggests that it is reasonable to view the responses at follow-up as relatively valid indicators of reasons for entrance. Nevertheless, keep in mind that the response differences might in part have reflected different experiences in the CCRC.

As might be expected, for both recent and longer-stay residents of extended and limited CCRCs the largest difference was in the proportion saying that the fees included nursing home care was important in their decision to move in. This was the case in both the comparison using the measure combining the *somewhat* and *very important* responses — hereinafter referred to as the response category *important* — and the comparison of persons saying the reason was very important in their decision to join the CCRC. As many as 90 percent of the recent residents of extended CCRCs said that fees including nursing home care was important in their decision; 84 percent said it was a very important reason. In contrast, a little under one third of the recent residents of limited CCRCs claimed this as an important reason, and only 22 percent said it was a very important reason. Similarly, among longer-stay residents, 90 percent of those in extended CCRCs said it was an important reason, but only 36 percent of those in limited CCRCs made this claim; as many as 85 percent of the longer-stay residents of extended CCRCs but only 26 percent of the longer-stay limited CCRC residents said it was a very important reason for entrance.

Correspondingly, the next largest difference between residents of extended and limited CCRCs, regardless of length of stay, was in whether residence was guaranteed even if their income would drop. Among recent residents, more than three quarters of those in extended CCRCs but less than half (47 percent) of those in limited CCRCs said that this was an important reason in their choice. As many as 67 percent of the recent residents of extended CCRCs but only 40 percent of their counterparts in limited CCRCs said it was a very important reason. Among longer-stay residents, almost three quarters of those in extended CCRCs compared with a little more than half of those in limited CCRCs said it was an important reason, dropping to 63 and 42 percent, respectively, saying that it was a very important reason for moving to the CCRC.

A system for handling medical emergencies was high on the list of attractive attributes regardless of the type of CCRC or resident's date of entrance. It was one of the two features specified by more than 85 percent of all four groups as important in their decision to move to the CCRC, and it was the only reason specified as very important by well over 85 percent of the recent residents of extended and limited CCRCs and more than 80 percent of the longer-stay residents. Clearly, most of the residents who considered this an important reason thought it was *very* important. At the same time, significantly more residents of extended than of limited CCRCs considered this important (96 and 90 percent, respectively, of the recent entrants of extended and limited CCRCs and 93 and 87 percent, respectively, of the longer-stay residents). Although the difference between longer-stay residents of the two types of CCRC remained significant when the *very important* responses were compared (89 percent of the longer-stay residents in extended CCRCs and 81 percent of those in limited CCRCs), the difference between recent residents in the two types of CCRC who said it was very important no longer met the criteria for statistical significance (91 percent of the extended and 86 percent of the limited CCRC residents).

Having a nice apartment — the second characteristic specified as important by more than 85 percent of all four groups — was high on the list of attractive features, with no significant difference between residents of extended and limited CCRCs, regardless of the length of stay or measure (important or very important) used. But the percentages dropped considerably when the *very important* responses were compared, particularly for the residents of extended CCRCs. Nevertheless, the percent who said that having a nice apartment was very important remained high — 68 percent of the longer-stay extended CCRC residents and more than 70 percent in the remaining groups.

Having extensive common areas also appears to be an attractive feature for recent and longer-stay residents in both types of CCRC. More than 70 percent in each of the groups said that this was at least somewhat important in their decision to move to the CCRC, with no significant differences in the responses of residents of extended and limited CCRCs. At the same time, only a minority in each group said that it was a very important reason for joining the CCRC; in this instance, significantly fewer of the recent residents of extended CCRCs (35 percent) than of limited CCRCs (43 percent) said that it was very important.

Other aspects of the environment — high-quality image/decor and location — were also considered important by more than three quarters of each of the comparison groups, regardless of their length of stay. However, significantly fewer of the recent residents of limited (79 percent) than of extended CCRCs (86 percent) felt that image/decor was important. Considerably fewer residents in each of the groups considered image/decor or location to be a very important reason for joining the CCRC. The percent in each group claiming image/decor to be a very important reason varied between 49 and 56 percent, with no significant differences between extended and limited CCRC residents. A larger percent in each of the groups said that location of the CCRC was a very important reason, in this case varying between 66 and 71 percent, with no significant differences between residents in the two types of CCRC.

A large number of all sample residents felt that the availability of nursing home and personal care services and ancillary IADL services (i.e., housekeeping, meals in the dining room, and available transportation) was an important reason for moving to the CCRC. In general, whether in comparisons of *important* or *very important* responses, residents of extended CCRCs were more likely than those of limited CCRCs to consider long-term care and ancillary IADL services important.

Transportation was the only service for which the difference in importance between residents in the two types of CCRC was significant only for the longer-stay residents; but even here, the difference between recent extended and limited CCRC residents was in the same direction. However, of the three ancillary services, transportation was considered important or very important by the fewest residents, regardless of group. Only a minority of residents in each group thought it was a very important reason for their joining the community, although significantly more of the longer-stay residents of extended CCRCs (48 percent) than of limited CCRCs (29 percent) thought so.

Well over a majority in each of these groups considered the availability of both nursing home and personal care services very important. Of the two long-term care services, a higher proportion in both extended and limited CCRCs, regardless of length of residence, considered the availability of a nursing home very important in their decision to move to the CCRC. As many as 89 and 73 percent of the recent residents of extended and limited CCRCs, respectively, considered the CCRC nursing home very important compared with 80 and 66 percent, respectively, of the recent residents of extended and limited CCRCs who said that personal care services were very important. Similarly, 92 and 71 percent of the longer-stay residents of extended and limited CCRCs, respectively, said that the availability of a nursing home was very important; 81 percent of the longer-stay extended CCRC residents and 58 percent of the limited CCRC residents said that personal care services were very important.

One other type of service was probed which was perhaps particularly relevant to persons who had formerly lived in a private home: maintenance and yard work done. More than three quarters of all groups said that this was an important consideration, and a majority in each group said it was very important. For this service, only the difference between longer-stay extended and limited CCRC residents who said it was an important reason was significant (85 and 77 percent, respectively); but when the *very important* responses were compared, only the difference between recent extended and limited CCRC residents was significant (64 and 54 percent, respectively).

Finally, a sizable majority of each group considered security/safety an important reason for entrance, but residents of extended CCRCs were significantly more likely to consider it so (81 and 62 percent, respectively, of the recent residents of extended and limited CCRCs and 75 and 68 percent, respectively, of the longer-stay residents). Except for recent residents of limited CCRCs, a majority of residents in each of the groups responded that security/safety was a very important reason; but using this measure, the difference between residents in the two types of CCRC in the percent who responded *very important* was significant only for recent residents (59 percent of the extended and 47 percent of the limited CCRC residents).[6]

Reasons-for-Entrance Scales

Factor analysis of the baseline and follow-up reasons revealed five distinct sets of questions: two sets from baseline and three from follow-up. Two reasons asked at follow-up (one pertaining to location and one to transportation) did not meet the minimum criteria for inclusion in any of the sets (i.e., the loadings of each of these items on each of the five factors were considerably less than 0.4). We constructed five scales (indices) based on these findings, one for each of the identified sets.

For the two scales involving baseline interview questions, each resident's score was the number of reasons in the set that was claimed as a reason for having chosen that type of retirement housing.

1. The *location scale* was a four-point scale (potential scores ranging from 0 to 3) based on three reasons concerning location and the people living at the CCRC: desirability of the apartment or location, wanting to be with people like oneself, and proximity to friends/relatives or a familiar area.

2. The *planning scale* was a six-point scale (scores from 0 to 5) based on five reasons addressing current and future protective needs: access to needed services now and in the future, protection features guaranteed in the contract, compensation for the absence or potential absence of helpers, avoidance of pressure or demands on family or friends, and guaranteed ability to live within one's means (protection of assets/independence).

For the three scales derived from questions asked at follow-up, we probed the importance of each reason, and the resident made a choice from three alternative responses: *very important* (scored as 2), *somewhat important* (scored as 1), or *not important* (scored as 0). For these scales, each resident's score was the sum of his or her responses to the questions in the scale, resulting in:

6. In general, the response patterns of recent and longer-stay residents within each type of CCRC were very similar. However, a higher percent of recent than of longer-stay residents of limited CCRCs said that availability of nursing home and personal care services was an important reason for their moving into the CCRC. For residents of extended CCRCs, a higher percentage of recent than of longer-stay residents said that security/safety was important in their decision.

3. The *IADL and environmental services scale*, a nine-point scale (scores from 0 to 8), was based on reasons concerning two IADL and two environmental services: housekeeping, availability of meals in the dining room, maintenance and yard work done, and security/safety provided.

4. The *health and financial concerns scale* was an eleven-point scale (scores from 0 to 10) based on five issues concerning emergency and long-term care, functional and medical health and related financial issues: a system for handling medical emergencies, availability of a nursing home, availability of personal care services, inclusion of nursing home care in the fees, and guaranteed residence even if income drops.

5. The *housing ambiance scale* was a seven-point scale (scores from 0 to 6) based on three questions dealing with the physical features of the CCRC: extent of common areas, quality of image and decor, and a attractiveness of the apartment unit.

The planning scale had an unacceptably low standardized alpha reliability (0.45), but we will present it anyway for descriptive purposes.[7] Since the scales contained different numbers of questions and therefore different metrics, we computed another score. For each scale, we divided the summed score by the maximum score possible for that scale; we referred to this as the *proportions score*. We converted to proportions to provide a basis for comparing the relative importance among the five reason domains as well as differences between the residents of the two types of facility. Table 2.5 depicts the mean proportion for each scale for recent and longer-stay residents of extended and limited CCRCs.

Clearly, health and financial concerns were most important for recent residents of extended CCRCs. Planning, IADL and environmental services, housing ambiance, and location followed, in that order. For recent residents of limited CCRCs, planning was most important, with housing ambiance, location, health and financial concerns, and IADL and environmental services following, in that order.

Residents of extended CCRCs appeared to have been much more concerned (than were residents of limited CCRCs) about medical/long-term care issues and were more likely to have chosen a CCRC in which those features were included as part of the contract. Based on the IADL and environmental services scale, they also apparently felt that the avail-

7. Using the combined samples for these computations, the standardized alpha reliabilities for each of the scales were as follows: location, 0.561; planning, 0.451; IADL/environmental services, 0.776; health and financial concerns, 0.699; and housing ambiance, 0.673.

Table 2.5 Proportions scales: Reasons for choosing the CCRC mean scale scores of residents by type of CCRC

Scales (higher score, more important)	Recent		Longer-stay	
	Extended (N = 281)	Limited (N = 220)	Extended (N = 549)	Limited (N = 579)
Location	0.51	0.65*	0.47	0.61*
Planning[a]	0.76	0.75	0.70	0.72
IADL and environmental services	0.73	0.58*	0.72	0.63*
Health and financial concerns	0.85	0.63*	0.86	0.61*
Housing ambiance	0.68	0.69	0.69	0.69

Note. The scores depicted in this table are mean scores for each of the subgroups on these five proportion scales. See the text for a description of how an individual's score on each of the scales was constructed. For comparisons between residents of extended and limited CCRCs, separately for recent and longer-stay residents, an asterisk to the right of the column depicting the mean score for residents of limited type CCRCs for a particular scale indicates that the difference between the two groups was statistically significant at the < 0.05 probability level; if no asterisk appears, the difference between the two groups was not considered statistically significant.

[a]Only one instance was found in which there was a significant difference between recent and longer-stay residents, whether of extended or limited type CCRCs: in extended CCRCs, planning was significantly more important to recent than to longer-stay residents. It must be kept in mind, however, that this was the only scale with an unacceptable standardized alpha reliability.

ability of such services was more important than did residents of limited CCRCs. The recent residents of limited CCRCs appeared to have been more concerned than their extended CCRC counterparts with the housing itself and with the people living there, although these were not the most important concerns for either group of residents.

The preference patterns of the longer-stay residents were very similar to those of the recent entrants. The same-scale differences were statistically different, and the ordering of importance among the scales within the CCRCs was the same. Health and financial concerns were again most important for residents of extended CCRCs, and housing ambiance and location again were relatively unimportant. For residents of limited CCRCs, planning and housing ambiance were most important, and health and financial concerns were relatively unimportant. The major difference was that the IADL/environmental services appeared to be slightly more important for longer-stay residents in limited CCRCs than for the more recent residents.

Health and financial concerns were most important for residents of extended CCRCs, and housing ambiance and location were relatively unimportant. For residents of limited CCRCs, planning and housing ambiance were most important, and health and financial concerns were relatively unimportant. Perhaps the larger apparent importance that the longer-stay rather than recent residents attached to these services reflected in part the increasing need for supportive services on the part of the longer-stay residents rather than an initial difference in their reasons for entrance.

The Residents: Conclusions and Insights

A comparison of the entrance characteristics of recent and longer-stay residents of the two types of facility yields insights regarding the CCRC marketplace. Specifically,

- The average age of entrance seems to be increasing, both for extended and limited CCRCs.
- More couples are moving into both types of CCRC.
- For limited CCRCs in particular, there appears to be an indication of an expansion of educational status groups considering entering limited CCRCs. Although the difference between recent and longer-stay residents of extended facilities is less clear, it appears that a similar expansion of educational groups interested in extended CCRCs may be emerging.

In some ways, residents of limited CCRCs are becoming more like the residents of extended CCRCs, suggesting the potential for an expanding market for limited CCRCs. Specifically,

- Although the population was largely Protestant in all samples, this was the case for significantly more of the longer-stay limited than extended CCRC residents. There were fewer Protestants, proportionately similar to their counterparts in extended CCRCs, among recent residents of limited CCRCs.
- In addition, although significantly fewer of the longer-stay residents of limited than extended facilities had learned about the CCRCs from friends, neighbors, relatives, and their church (informal sources), a significantly larger percent of recent residents of limited than of extended facilities had learned about the CCRC from informal sources.

Although only a minority of residents entered from another retirement community (very few from other CCRCs), it appears that more of those moving to extended than to limited CCRCs have had prior experience living in an age-segregated (older adult) community. Other retirement communities that have no pooled-risk features either for nursing home care or supportive services may represent a particularly good market for organizations planning to develop extended CCRC facilities.

Findings regarding the proportions of recent and longer-stay residents who had never been married at baseline are illuminating.[8] Although no more than 15 percent of any group had never married (were single) by baseline, considerably more (at least 1.75 times as many) of the longer-stay than recent residents had never married (and the difference between recent and longer-stay residents within each type of CCRC was statistically significant).[9] Previously, CCRCs appeared to have been particularly attractive to single (never married) elderly people; but the proportion of single persons among the recent residents is considerably less and is now similar to the 1980 national population of single persons 75 years and older (see Chapter 1).

The data about the number of children at baseline, regardless of the type of community or length of residence, have implications for the informal support system. CCRC residents in general appeared to have had only a small number of living children, with an average of fewer than 1.4 in any of the groups. This, coupled with the fact that on average one third or fewer of these children were nearby, indicates that these CCRC residents were to a large extent not in a position to call on children for informal help even if they had wanted to do so.

Analysis of entrance and baseline characteristics as well as reasons for entrance point to both similarities and differences between the residents of extended and limited CCRCs. For the most part, entrance and baseline characteristics and reasons for entrance of extended and limited CCRC residents followed the same patterns, even when significant differences between groups occurred. If a characteristic was predominant in one of the samples, it was usually predominant in the remaining samples. As examples, in each sample there was a high proportion of females; a scarcity of foreign born residents; a small number with a child within a one-hour drive; a large proportion with income from investments; a majority who said that having protective features guaranteed in the CCRC contract was a reason that applied to them; and a large majority who said that a nice apartment unit and availability of a nursing home and personal care services were very important in their decision to move to the CCRC.

The largest difference between extended and limited CCRC residents, regardless of the length of stay, was in educational status, with

8. This cannot be considered an entrance characteristic since some persons, the longer-stay residents in particular, who had never been married at entrance might have married in the interim.

9. The larger percent of longer-stay persons within each type of CCRC who had never married may in part account for the smaller mean number of living children and the smaller mean number of children within a one-hour drive of the longer-stay residents.

residents of extended CCRCs consistently reaching a higher level of education (both in the percent who were college graduates and in the average number of years of education). Although the differences between extended and limited CCRC residents and in where persons lived before entrance were not as stark as educational status, for both recent and longer-stay residents consistently more residents of limited CCRCs were living in a private house, but, as indicated above, fewer moved to the CCRC from another retirement community.

Even though well over 90 percent in each of the sample groups had income from investments, a small but consistently significantly larger proportion of residents of extended than limited CCRCs had income from this source. However, a much higher percentage of extended than limited CCRC residents drew upon interest, whether from savings, investments, or trust funds, to pay the monthly fee. Although from the data at hand there is no way of knowing why this was so, questions such as the following can be raised: Is the mix of sources of income different for residents in the two types of CCRC (e.g., Do extended residents have more money in trust funds and/or savings)? Are residents of limited CCRCs more dependent on pensions than on interest from savings, investments, and trust funds for their income? Do they have less money in savings, investments, and/or trust funds? To what extent do the generally larger monthly fees of extended CCRCs impact differentially on the necessity to draw upon interest from these sources to pay the monthly fee? As indicated by the much larger proportions of extended CCRC residents who spend money regularly on outside entertainment, do differences in life style between extended CCRC residents necessitate drawing upon rather than piling up the interest from these sources? Does the certainty that they will not need excessive amounts of money to cover the costs of potential long-term care (nursing home services) enter the picture (e.g., are they willing to spend money regularly on outside entertainment rather than saving for future needs)?

With one notable exception, close to 50 percent or more of the residents in both types of CCRC, regardless of length of stay, said that each of the reasons queried in the baseline and follow-up interviews applied to them or was somewhat or very important. Although the percentages dropped for the questions concerning the degree of importance, for the most part sizable proportions close to 50 percent or more in both types of CCRC considered the reason very important in their decision to join the CCRC. Nevertheless, consistent significant differences were found between residents in the two types of CCRC.

In line with what each type of CCRC offered, the largest and key difference between residents of extended and limited CCRCs was in the proportion who said that having nursing home care included in the fee was important in their decision to move to the CCRC. As many as 90 percent of both recent and longer-stay residents in extended facilities considered this an important reason for entrance, with 84 to 85 percent saying it was a very important reason. Of the recent residents in limited facilities, fewer than one third said it was important, dropping to 22 percent who said it was very important. Similar proportions were found for the longer-stay residents.

For residents of extended CCRCs the pooled risk for future costs of care and planning to maintain one's life style were also important as indicated by the next largest difference between residents of extended and limited CCRCs in their reasons for entrance: guaranteed residence even if their income would drop. Among recent residents, more than three quarters of those in extended CCRCs said this was an important reason, decreasing to more than two thirds who said it was a very important reason in their choice. Far fewer in limited CCRCs made this claim; 46 percent said it was important, and 40 percent said it was very important. There were comparable differences between the longer-stay residents in the two types of CCRC.

A large majority of residents in each type of facility said the availability of a nursing home was important; slightly fewer considered it very important. A large majority in each group also considered personal care services important. The percentage decreased relatively little for the extended CCRC residents but more so for limited CCRC residents, who said such services were very important reasons for their moving to the CCRC.

For the most part, the majority in each group also thought that supportive services — particularly meals and housekeeping — were important, but the proportions dropped considerably for the response *very important*. Clearly, IADL services were lower in priority than access to the nursing home and personal care.

A system for handling medical emergencies was high on the list of attractive features, regardless of the CCRC type or date of entrance, with a large majority considering it a very important reason for moving to the CCRC. Although less so than for handling medical emergencies, all groups felt that having a nice apartment was important, with large majorities considering it very important.

Reasons-for-entrance scale scores indicated distinct differences between the residents of extended and limited CCRCs. Residents of extended CCRCs consistently considered health and financial matters and IADL/environmental services more important than did residents of limited CCRCs. Residents of limited CCRCs consistently rated location as more important than did extended CCRC residents. For both recent and longer-stay residents, no differences were found on the scales measuring housing ambiance and planning.

The ordering of reasons was very different for the two groups of residents and was logically related to the features of the two types of CCRC. Residents of extended CCRCs appeared to have been much more concerned about medical/long-term care issues and therefore chose a CCRC in which those services were included as part of the contract. Both types of resident were concerned with planning issues. For residents of limited CCRCs, planning and housing ambiance were relatively most important, and health and financial concerns were relatively unimportant.

Similarities and differences in the responses to the individual items and scores on the reasons-for-entrance scales both point to the same conclusion: elderly persons entering these CCRCs tend to act rationally. Their reasons for selecting their CCRC are in line with the services that are offered.

THREE

Residents in the Light
of Their CCRC Experience

Comparisons of resident background characteristics and their reasons for entrance support the contention that extended and limited CCRCs may be particularly attractive to different types of people. In this chapter we will focus on the differences and similarities in the experiences and reactions of residents in these two types of CCRC. In particular, we examine:

- activities of residents, including use of CCRC leisure-time resources (amenities) and participation in activities before and after joining the CCRC;
- residents' attitudes and perceptions of the CCRC living arrangement;
- selected quality-of-life indices.

Samples, Data Sources, and Analyses

The samples used in the analyses we present in this chapter were the same as those used in Chapter 2 (comparing the characteristics of extended and limited CCRC residents at entrance and at baseline and the residents' reasons for entrance). These individuals were CCRC apartment dwellers[1] at baseline and had both baseline and follow-up interviews approximately sixteen months later. In all, these samples consisted of 281 recent residents from extended CCRCs, 220 recent residents from limited CCRCs, 549 longer-stay residents from extended CCRCs, and 579 longer-stay residents from limited CCRCs. As in Chapter 2, we compared residents of extended and limited CCRCs and completed separate analyses for recent and longer-stay residents.

To a large extent we derived the data for these analyses from in-depth follow-up interviews with residents. However, we also used data obtained from the baseline interview in selected multivariate analyses. We will present the interview questions or items/response categories in detail along with the findings.

---

1. Recall that independent living units (ILUs) could be apartments, town houses, or cottages. For the sake of convenience, we refer to ILUs as *apartments*.

Discriminant Function Analyses

In the search for covariates to employ in selected controlled comparisons of the outcomes that residents experienced, we used discriminant function analyses to identify a set of entrance and baseline characteristics which distinguished residents of extended and limited CCRCs.

Activities

We based our descriptions of and comparisons between activities of residents of extended and limited CCRCs on data we collected at follow-up about their use of five recreational facilities/programs (amenities) available in all of the study CCRCs as well as residents' participation in fifteen leisure-time activities. We addressed the residents' use of the individual amenities and participation in each of the activities (participation variables). We also constructed summary scales that counted the number of CCRC amenities the resident used; the activities in which the resident participated at the CCRC; the activities that the resident discontinued upon moving to the CCRC; and the activities in which the resident never participated, either before or after moving to the CCRC.

We employed the chi-square statistic to determine the level of significance of compared percentages of extended and limited CCRC residents using each CCRC amenity or participating or not in each of the fifteen activities. For each of the scales, we performed t-tests to determine the significance of differences between the mean scores of residents of extended and limited CCRCs. In addition, for two of the scales that measured the use of amenities and activity participation while a CCRC resident, we employed two-way analysis of variance (ANOVA) to examine interrelationships between scale scores and the baseline self-report of health, the type of CCRC, and the self-report of health by type of CCRC. We conducted similar analyses of interrelationships between scores on each of these scales and age, type of CCRC, and age by type of CCRC.

Residents' Attitudes and Perceptions of the CCRC Living Arrangement

The analyses focused on attitudes and perceptions at follow-up. As part of the in-depth follow-up interview, we asked residents about their perceptions of the CCRC living arrangement. We had asked four of these questions previously during the baseline interview.

We asked two sets of questions at follow-up only. One set, consisting of six questions, directly probed residents' opinions as to various features of the CCRC living arrangement. The second set, consisting of ten questions, probed their experience with the availability of services when needed. For each set of questions, we constructed a summary scale consisting of an index of general satisfaction, based on counts of positive responses to questions about the CCRC, and a service-availability index, based on the number of times each resident mentioned that a service, when needed, was unavailable. We used the t-test statistic to determine the significance of the difference between the mean responses of residents of extended and limited CCRCs, for both the individual items and the comparison of scale scores.[2]

For each of the four variables probed at both baseline and follow-up, we investigated attitudinal differences between residents of extended and limited CCRCs at both points in time (using t-tests) as well as with-in-sample attitudinal changes from baseline to follow-up (using paired t-tests). We also performed logistic regressions for ordinal categories with covariates to estimate what the differences in attitude would have been between the residents in extended and limited CCRCs at follow-up had the two samples been more alike at baseline. For each satisfaction variable, we used as covariates baseline characteristics identified through discriminant function analysis (described below), which differentiated residents in the two types of CCRC, and the baseline scores for that variable.

Selected Quality-of-Life Indices

We analyzed two quality-of-life indices, each consisting of questions that we asked during both the baseline and follow-up interviews. One index was a previously standardized scale, *attitude toward own aging*, an identified component of the larger Philadelphia Geriatric Center (PGC) Morale Scale (Morris and Sherwood 1975). The second index, a *quality-of-life scale*, was based on factor analysis we performed to find a cluster of variables which might yield a more meaningful composite score. (We will describe the items and scoring systems for each of these scales later.) The analytic procedures were the same as those for comparing the baseline and follow-up attitudes of extended and limited CCRC residents toward the CCRC living arrangement.

Discriminant Function Analyses

We performed a series of discriminant function analyses to identify variables for common use in selected controlled comparisons of follow-up status of residents in extended and limited CCRCs. We wanted variables that would take into account basic differences in the background characteristics of residents in these two types of CCRC. We performed

2. For clarity, in the text we present percentages on individual items. Therefore, we applied the chi-square statistic also to questions with dichotomous response categories, yielding essentially the same results.

each discriminant function analysis in this series separately for recent and longer-stay residents. In the initial discriminant function analyses, we used thirty-six variables: the thirteen entrance characteristics and twenty-three of the twenty-four characteristics derived from the baseline interview described in Tables 2.1 and 2.2[3] Appendix B, Table B1, presents the standardized canonical coefficients of the final discriminant functions differentiating between extended and limited CCRC residents.

Because there were many similarities between residents of the two types of CCRC, the final set of discriminant function analyses produced only a modest hit rate (i.e., successful prediction) of group membership: 72.1 percent for recent and 66.3 percent for longer-stay residents. We entered an identical set of thirteen variables into both equations as well as an additional two variables, income and the IADL index, into the discriminant function equation for longer-stay residents. For convenience, we used all fifteen as the set for controlled comparisons.

Six of the fifteen variables were entrance characteristics: education, religion (Protestant/not Protestant), whether or not the resident learned about the CCRC from informal sources, whether or not the resident visited other CCRCs before selecting the facility, home ownership before entering the CCRC, and whether the resident lived in a retirement community or other CCRC before moving to this CCRC. Three baseline demographic features were among these fifteen: income, whether or not the resident had income from investments, and number of living children. The remaining six included two functional status variables (the IADL index and level of self-sufficiency); two variables regarding resources drawn upon to finance the monthly fee (*interest* from savings, investments, and/or trust funds; *principal* from savings, trust funds, and/or proceeds from sale of property); and two additional variables involving financial concerns (how much out-of-pocket medical expense the resident incurred in the previous month above and beyond what was received from Medicare and/or health insurance and not including vacations and whether the resident spent money regularly for entertainment outside the home such as movies, plays, concerts, and sporting events).

Activities of CCRC Residents

Because a resident's actual use of available amenities and participation in activities most likely reflected leisure interests before entering the CCRC, his or her use of CCRC resources and activities might often be a

---

3. We omitted one of the educational variables discussed above. Specifically, because *college graduate* is a simple dichotomy derived from *educational level*, we used only the more inclusive educational variable in these analyses.

continuation of those interests. On the other hand, other factors might have contributed to nonparticipation — factors such as health and age, ease of access, encouragement to join activities by friends and neighbors, and attitudes and encouragement or discouragement by CCRC staff and community professionals.

Analyses of the age and the perceived health status and age of CCRC residents in relation to leisure-time activities can add to an understanding of the extent to which differences in these characteristics were related to resident activities. In addition, self-reported data about prior (before entering the CCRC) participation in the same recreational activities may shed some light on similarities and differences in the recreational orientation of residents of extended and limited CCRCs.

Use of CCRC Recreational Facilities/Programs

Of eight CCRC amenities that we probed systematically, five were available in all nineteen of the study CCRCs. These were: craft or activity room, health club or exercise classes, billiards or game room, library, and chapel. Resources that were not universally available were: commissary or coffee shop, swimming pool or spa, and tennis courts.

As shown in Table 3.1, the library was the facility used by the largest percentage of residents of all four samples (recent and longer-stay residents in extended and limited CCRCs). Health club/exercise classes were used by the smallest percentage of residents. This pattern of use crossed all four samples in terms of the rank order of percentages of users: library, chapel, crafts/activities room, game room, and health club/exercise classes. For both the recent and longer-stay samples, residents of extended CCRCs were significantly more likely than those of limited facilities to use the library and the chapel.

To examine further this area of resident behavior, we compared the mean scores of the scale measuring use of CCRC facilities (an average of the number of resources used by residents in each sample) for the residents in the two types of CCRC. Recent residents of extended CCRCs took advantage of significantly more of the CCRC leisure-time facilities and programs (averaging 2.10 out of the five amenities) than did residents of limited CCRCs (who averaged 1.86). The difference, however, was not significant for the longer-stay samples (averaging 2.21 and 2.09 for the residents of extended and limited CCRCs, respectively). The difference between recent but not longer-stay residents in these two types of CCRC suggests that it may have taken a little longer for residents of limited CCRCs to start using the facility amenities.

Alternatively, the observed differences between recent residents in the extended and limited communities may have been a function of

Table 3.1 Residents who made use of CCRC resources, by length of residence and type of CCRC

	Recent		Longer-stay	
	Extended (N = 281)	Limited (N = 220)	Extended (N = 549)	Limited (N = 579)
	%	%	%	%
Craft/activities room	3.4	30.1	36.2	39.7
Health club classes	19.9	25.5	18.6	18.8
Game room	26.3	29.5	27.5	26.4
Library	79.0*	64.1	80.3*	74.8
Chapel	50.9*	37.3	58.3*	49.4

Note. An asterisk indicates that the difference between residents of extended and limited CCRCs was statistically significant at $p < 0.05$.

differences in case mix, broadly defined here as distributions of resident characteristics in general rather than limited to medical and long-term care needs. Differences in age and perceived health between residents in these two types of facility suggest that this might be the case. As we discussed in Chapter 2, in the comparisons of both recent and longer-stay residents, those in extended CCRCs perceived themselves as healthier than their counterparts in limited CCRCs. Furthermore, longer-stay residents in limited CCRCs were older than their counterparts in extended CCRCs. For example, as many as 40 percent, compared with 33 percent of the extended CCRC residents, were 85 years of age or older. Although not statistically significant, the age difference was in the same direction for recent residents. Given these differences in age and perceived health, we investigated more closely the interrelationships between these variables and the use of the five amenities.

Using a two-way ANOVA—health by type of CCRC—for both recent and longer-stay resident samples, we found a significant health effect: the healthier the resident, the greater the use of the available amenities (see Appendix B, Table B2). But controlling for health variability, we found no difference between residents in limited and extended CCRCs, for either the recent or longer-stay samples. The difference in the use of CCRC amenities appears to be a function of differences in the health levels and variables related to health of the two sets of residents and *not* attributable to differences between the extended and limited facilities.[4]

4. Of the residents in excellent health, those of limited CCRCs, regardless of their length of stay, used slightly more resources than residents of extended CCRCs. However,

An analysis of interrelationships among age, type of CCRC, and use of CCRC leisure-time resources produced very similar findings (see Appendix B, Table B3). There was a significant relationship between the average use of CCRC leisure-time resources and residents' age for both the recent and the longer-stay residents; younger residents were more likely than older residents to have used more CCRC amenities. Again, as with the perceived health variable, there was no type-of-CCRC effect; observed differences in the use of leisure-time resources appeared to be a function of differences in the characteristics (health, age, and related variables) of the samples of residents rather than attributable to the facilities.

Participation in Leisure-Time Activities

By the time of the follow-up interview, even the recent sample members had more than a year of experience at the CCRC. We asked residents about their participation, both before and after coming to the CCRC, in fifteen types of leisure-time activity. We asked them whether they now or had ever attended, engaged in, belonged to, or participated in concerts, theater, lectures, academic classes, sporting events, movies, church groups, social clubs, community service, volunteer activity, support groups, family gatherings, travel, gathering with friends, or hobbies.

The response categories differentiated among persons who had participated in the activity only before moving to the CCRC, those who had participated before and continued to do so after becoming a CCRC resident, those who had participated in the activity only after becoming a CCRC resident, and those who had never participated in the activity. As shown in Tables 3.2 and 3.3, there was considerable variation across the fifteen activities for all four categories of participation (only before, before and after, only since, and never) for both the recent and the longer-stay samples.

Participation in Activities while a CCRC Resident. There was much diversity in the activities in which residents of both types of CCRC participated. At the same time, there was considerable similarity in the pattern of participation across both types of CCRC samples, regardless

---

among those in good or fair/poor health, residents of extended CCRC used more CCRC resources than did residents of limited CCRCs. In the two-way ANOVA comparisons involving age, type of CCRC, and average score on the scale measuring the use of CCRC amenities, the same was the case for recent residents. For each age category for the longer-stay residents, the average score for extended CCRC residents was slightly higher than the score for limited CCRC residents (see Appendix B, Table B1).

Table 3.2 Recent residents who stated that they participated in activity, by type of CCRC

Activity	Extended CCRC (N = 281)				Limited CCRC (N = 220)			
	Only before	Before and after	Only since	Never	Only before	Before and after	Only since	Never
	%	%	%	%	%	%	%	%
Concerts	13.0	70.8	2.9	13.4	19.5	60.5	2.3	17.7
Theater	27.4	56.0	1.4	15.2	30.7	53.0	1.9	14.4
Lectures	15.6	69.9	4.3	10.1	17.8	57.0	3.7	21.5
Academic classes	31.4	14.1	1.8	52.7	28.5	7.9	0.5	63.1
Sporting events	37.9	19.5	0.7	41.9	36.3	17.2	0.5	46.9
Movies	34.7	52.0	1.1	12.3	31.2	33.5	0.9	34.4
Church groups	25.6	57.8	0.7	15.9	23.7	60.0	0.0	16.3
Social clubs	27.8	39.0	0.7	32.5	24.2	30.2	0.0	45.6
Community service	26.4	26.0	1.1	46.6	24.7	30.7	0.5	44.2
Volunteer activity	19.5	50.9	5.4	24.2	21.3	50.5	3.7	24.5
Support groups	2.9	9.7	2.5	84.8	4.2	5.6	0.9	89.3
Family gatherings	14.8	82.3	0.0	2.9	10.7	76.7	1.4	11.2
Travel	23.8	72.6	0.0	3.6	28.7	63.4	2.3	5.6
Gathering with friends	8.3	89.5	0.4	1.8	12.0	87.0	0.0	0.9
Hobbies	13.0	79.8	0.4	6.9	16.2	77.8	0.5	5.6

of length of residence. More than 50 percent of both the recent and the longer-stay residents in both extended and limited CCRCs participated in nine of these activities: concerts, theater, lectures, church groups, volunteer activity, family gatherings, travel, gatherings with friends, and hobbies. Gathering with friends ranked first, and family gatherings ranked either second or third in all four samples. Movies, social clubs, community services, sporting events, academic classes, and support groups were the six least popular activities for all four samples and were ranked in exactly the same order, tenth to fifteenth, respectively.

Despite similar profiles, we found significant differences in CCRC resident participation for seven of these activities. Both recent and longer-stay residents of extended facilities were more likely than their counterparts in limited CCRCs to attend lectures and movies. Of the longer-stay samples, residents of extended CCRCs were significantly more likely than those of limited CCRCs to participate in family gatherings and gatherings with friends. However, a significantly larger proportion of longer-stay residents of limited CCRCs than of extended CCRCs participated in volunteer activities.

The summary scale score of participation in activities while a CCRC resident included continued participation in a pre-CCRC activity after

Table 3.3 Longer-stay residents who stated that they participated in activity, by type of CCRC

Activity	Extended CCRC (N = 549)				Limited CCRC (N = 579)			
	Only before	Before and after	Only since	Never	Only before	Before and after	Only since	Never
	%	%	%	%	%	%	%	%
Concerts	17.2	74.8	3.6	4.5	24.6	62.6	2.3	10.5
Theater	30.0	60.8	2.4	6.8	30.6	56.8	1.1	11.6
Lectures	10.1	72.2	5.4	8.2	18.0	59.6	6.4	16.0
Academic classes	33.5	7.5	1.3	57.7	35.5	9.4	0.5	54.5
Sporting events	36.0	9.4	0.0	54.7	45.6	14.8	0.7	38.9
Movies	32.7	54.4	1.3	11.6	39.3	42.0	0.7	18.0
Church groups	27.7	56.4	0.7	15.2	20.9	66.1	0.2	12.8
Social clubs	36.5	32.4	0.9	30.1	36.3	28.6	0.7	34.5
Community service	29.2	19.4	1.5	49.9	38.1	27.1	0.0	34.8
Volunteer activity	22.0	53.3	6.9	17.8	19.1	60.5	5.7	14.7
Support groups	4.2	3.6	3.2	89.0	2.2	4.0	1.3	92.6
Family gatherings	15.7	77.0	0.6	6.7	20.3	68.6	0.5	10.5
Travel	29.9	68.2	0.6	1.3	28.7	67.6	0.7	3.0
Gathering with friends	3.2	96.1	0.0	0.7	11.2	87.5	0.2	1.1
Hobbies	13.7	80.3	0.2	5.8	17.1	76.4	0.2	6.3

moving to the CCRC as well as activities begun only after moving to the CCRC. Recent residents of extended CCRCs participated as residents in an average of 8.01 of these fifteen activities, whereas residents of limited CCRCs participated in an average of 7.15. For longer-stay residents, the mean scores on this scale were 7.77 and 7.29 for residents of extended and limited CCRCs, respectively. In both instances, residents of extended CCRCs participated while they were residents of the CCRC in significantly more activities than did the residents of limited CCRCs (see Appendix B, Table B4).

Discontinuation of Activities in Which the Resident Participated before Moving to the CCRC. Residents of both types of CCRC appeared to have ceased participating in a substantial number of leisure-time activities. There were no differences between the recent residents of extended and limited CCRCs in the average number of the activities in which they participated only before joining the CCRC. Both discontinued, on average, approximately three activities after entering the CCRC (averaging 3.17 for residents of extended CCRCs and 3.22 for those of limited CCRCs). But the findings for the longer-stay samples are quite different. The residents of limited CCRCs discontinued, on the average, more (3.75) activities than did the residents of extended CCRCs (3.32) (see Appendix B, Table B4).

CCRC residents nevertheless appeared to be an active group. But when compared with the activities reported for an earlier period of their lives, there was a considerable reduction in overall participation by the residents in both types of CCRC. Tables 3.2 and 3.3 reveal that the CCRCs did not elicit much participation in activities different from those in which the residents had participated before entering the CCRC. The percentages of *only since* participation were quite small. From this perspective, neither type of CCRC appeared to have had much of a positive effect on increasing the number of residents' leisure-time activities from their former level. An examination of the *only since* columns of Tables 3.2 and 3.3 reveals that these losses, if we may call them that, were not in any way made up by new participation in these activities (i.e., by residents who had not participated in the activities before coming to the CCRC but did so afterward).

For example, about one fourth or more of the residents in all four samples discontinued participation in church groups; less than 1 percent of former nonparticipants became new members of church groups. Large proportions of the residents who had previously attended movies discontinued this behavior. Almost no one who had not previously attended movies began to do so after coming to the CCRC (less than 2 percent in each of the four samples). Participation in sporting events was an even more extreme example; two thirds or more who had previously attended sporting events ceased to do so after coming to the CCRC.

Nonparticipation in Activities before and after CCRC Residence. There was great diversity across the fifteen activities in terms of the percent who had never participated in the activity either before coming to or while at the facility. As many as 80 percent or more of all four samples had never participated in support groups. Approximately 50 percent had never participated in academic classes (as a leisure-time activity), and half or slightly fewer had never participated in sporting events or community service. After support groups and academic classes, the largest percentages of recent residents of both extended and limited CCRCs stated that they had never participated in community service, sporting events, and social clubs. At the other extreme, almost none claimed to have never participated in gatherings with friends — fewer than twenty residents of the total of more than fifteen hundred in the four samples. Very few of the residents of either type of CCRC or in either of the two length-of-stay resident groups had never participated in the activities of travel and hobbies.

We found a significant difference between the means for the recent residents of the two types of CCRC on the scale constructed by counting for each resident the number of activities in which that resident had never participated. The recent residents of limited CCRCs had never participated in an average of 4.3 activities. The mean for the residents of extended CCRCs was 3.59. There was no difference for the longer-stay residents (see Appendix B, Table B4); of these fifteen activities, the average number in which residents of limited CCRCs had never participated was 3.47; and the number was 3.49 for residents of extended CCRCs.

Perceived (Self-Reported) Health at Baseline and Participation while a CCRC Resident. Since there was a significant baseline difference between the recent residents in extended and limited CCRCs in perceived health, we performed additional analyses of the extent of participation in leisure-time activities (using the two-way ANOVA statistical technique) to determine whether there were significant interrelationships among health rating, type of CCRC, and participation in leisure-time activities while a resident (see Appendix B, Table B5).

Findings from this analysis indicate that the better the health rating, the greater the number of activities in which sample members participated while a CCRC resident, regardless of length of stay. However, the mean differences between participation scores of residents in the two types of CCRC were similar across the health status subgroups (i.e., in more technical terms, interactions between health rating and type of CCRC were not statistically significant). In other words, for both the recent and longer-stay samples, differences in health status did not account for the observed differences in participation in leisure-time activities between residents in these extended and limited CCRCs. In fact, both for recent and longer-stay residents, residents of extended CCRCs participated in significantly more activities while residents of the CCRC than did residents of limited CCRCs.

Age at Baseline and Participation. Because we observed a significant baseline age difference between residents in these two types of CCRC, we performed a similar analysis to determine whether there were significant interrelationships among age, type of CCRC, and participation in leisure-time activities while a resident.

Findings from these ANOVAs indicate that the mean differences between participation scores of residents in the two types of CCRC were similar across the age subgroups (i.e., interactions between age at baseline and type of CCRC were not statistically significant). In general, then, for both the recent and longer-stay samples, the difference between the age distributions did not account for the observed differences between residents in extended and limited types of CCRC in participation in leisure-time activities (see Appendix B, Table B6).

Residents' Attitudes and Perceptions of the CCRC Living Arrangement

We asked sample members questions that dealt either directly or indirectly with their satisfaction with the CCRC living arrangement. First at baseline and then again at follow-up we probed a number of specific attitudes and one about the residents' general attitudes toward the CCRC. We asked additional questions at follow-up only, with a focus on the residents' perceptions of specific services. Although data gathered at both interviews enabled us to analyze changes in satisfaction, keep in mind that baseline attitudes of recent entrants were often based on the experience of only a few weeks of actual residence. Follow-up attitudes and perceptions, however, reflected a minimum of one year of experience for all sample members. Therefore, this analysis focused primarily on satisfaction at follow-up. When they were available, however, we considered baseline attitudes in controlled analyses regarding outcome at follow-up and changes during the study period.

Questions Asked at Follow-Up Only

One set of questions probed directly opinions relating to various features of the CCRC living arrangement. Another set probed the experience of sample members regarding the availability of services when needed. We inferred dissatisfaction with a service if a resident had needed a particular service but had been unable to get it.

Satisfaction with CCRC. The following questions probed opinions directly relating to the resident's satisfaction with the CCRC:

- Are you satisfied with your housing?
- Are you satisfied with the care provided at the health center (i.e., the CCRC nursing home)?
- Thinking it over now, was it a good decision to move to the CCRC?
- Did the CCRC meet your expectations?
- All things considered, do you think the cost of living at the CCRC is a good value?
- Would you recommend the CCRC to others?

These questions called for a *yes* (indicating satisfaction) or a *no* (indicating dissatisfaction) response. However, a sizable minority of the sample members said that they had no opinion regarding the care provided at the health center (28 percent of the recent and 19 percent of the longer-stay residents of extended CCRCs and 46 percent and 32 percent of the recent and longer-stay residents of limited CCRCs).[5] We considered a *yes* answer to indicate distinct satisfaction, a *no opinion* answer to mean that the respondent was at least not dissatisfied, and a *no* response to indicate distinct dissatisfaction. We scored the responses to this question (1 = yes; 2 = no opinion; and 3 = no) and performed *t*-tests on these data and the remaining five questions (with 1 = yes and 2 = no) to determine the significance of the difference between residents of extended and limited CCRCs.

Table 3.4 describes the percentage within each sample expressing satisfaction with various aspects of the CCRC. Because of the large percentages who voiced no opinion as to care in the CCRC health center, we present two figures: the percentage of the total sample who said they were satisfied and the percentage of those with opinions who were satisfied.

Large percentages (85 percent or more) of all four samples were satisfied with the housing and with the cost of living at the CCRC, thought that moving to the CCRC had been a good decision, and would recommend the CCRC to others. At least 92 percent of all groups were satisfied with their housing, and 95 percent or more said it had been a good decision to move to the CCRC. More than 91 percent of the recent and 93 percent of the longer-stay residents of extended CCRCs thought that the cost of living at the CCRC was a good value; 89 percent of the recent but only 86 percent of the longer-stay residents of limited CCRCs (significantly less than their counterparts in extended CCRCs) thought so. Smaller percentages felt that the CCRC was meeting expectations or were distinctly satisfied with the health center. Nevertheless, even here a large majority of longer-stay residents in extended CCRCs (87 percent) and sizable majorities in the remaining groups were satisfied that the CCRC did meet expectations (78 and 61 percent, respectively, of recent residents of extended and limited CCRCs and 70 percent of longer-stay residents of limited CCRCs). Also, if we excluded from the samples those who did not voice an opinion, as many as 89 percent of the recent and 91 percent of the longer-stay residents in extended facilities and 90 percent of the recent and 82 percent of the longer-stay residents in limited CCRCs expressed satisfaction with the health center.

For both the recent and the longer-stay samples, significantly (*t*-test) more residents of extended CCRCs than those of limited CCRCs would

5. In all, the sizes of the samples expressing an opinion (i.e., they said *yes* or *no*) were 202 recent residents of extended and 120 of limited CCRCs and 447 longer-stay residents of extended and 394 of limited CCRCs.

Table 3.4 Recent and longer-stay residents expressing satisfaction with various aspects of CCRC, by type of CCRC

Variable[a]	Recent		Longer-stay	
	Extended (N = 281)	Limited (N = 220)	Extended (N = 549)	Limited (N = 579)
	%	%	%	%
Housing	95.4	92.7	95.4	91.9
Health care center (total Ns)	63.7	45.5	74.0	55.6
Of those expressing an opinion[b]	88.6	90.0	90.8	81.7
Decision to move to CCRC	96.1	95.0	98.9	94.8
CCRC meeting expectation	78.3	61.4	86.7	70.3
Cost of living at CCRC	91.1	88.6	93.1	86.2
Recommend CCRC to others	97.5	90.5	95.1	94.5
Satisfaction scale	Mean scores			
Sum of positive responses (0 to 6)	5.20	4.77[c]	5.37	4.75[c]

[a]The t-test statistic was used to test the significance of differences, scoring all but satisfaction with care provided at the health center as 1 = yes, 2 = no; and for care at the health center: 1 = yes, 2 = no opinion, and 3 = no. Significant differences between recent residents in the two types of CCRC — both in favor of the extended CCRCs — were observed for satisfaction with care at the health center (p = 0.05) and whether they would recommend (p ≤ 0.05) the CCRC to others. For longer-stay residents, significant differences were found for all six items, all in favor of the extended CCRCs except for satisfaction with housing (p ≤ 0.01); all differences were significant at p ≤ 0.001.

[b]The samples expressing an opinion were: 202 recent residents of extended and 120 of limited CCRCs; 447 longer-stay residents of extended and 394 of limited CCRCs.

[c]Significant differences between scale scores of residents of extended and limited CCRCs were statistically significant at p ≤ 0.001.

have recommended the facility to others and were satisfied with the health center. Significantly more of the longer-stay residents of extended CCRCs than of limited CCRCs were satisfied with their housing, thought that it had been a good decision to move to the CCRC, thought the CCRC was meeting expectations, and were satisfied with the cost of living at the CCRC.

Summary Measure of Satisfaction. An index of general satisfaction was constructed for each resident which consisted of the number of favorable (*yes*) responses to the six questions. The average number of *yes* responses was significantly higher for residents of extended CCRCs than for the residents of limited CCRCs. This was true for both recent and longer-stay residents. For recent residents, the mean score was 5.20 for residents of extended CCRCs and 4.77 for residents of limited CCRCs.

For longer-stay residents, the mean scores were 5.37 and 4.75, respectively (see Table 3.4).

Slightly more than 50 percent of the recent residents of extended CCRCs responded favorably to all six questions compared with slightly more than 35 percent of the residents of limited CCRCs. The findings for the longer-stay samples were similar. In fact, the difference between the samples from the two types of CCRC was even greater: 60 percent of the residents of extended CCRCs compared with 40 percent of those of limited CCRCs responded favorably to all six questions.

A clear conclusion is that residents of extended CCRCs were more satisfied in general about their CCRC experience than were residents of limited CCRCs. We should reemphasize, however, that both recent and longer-stay residents of both types of CCRC appeared to be very satisfied with their facility.

Service Availability. At follow-up, we asked residents whether there had been a time that they had needed services and had been unable to get them at the CCRC. We recorded their responses about the needed availability of the following ten categories: light housework, chores, transportation, shopping/errands, meal preparation, personal care, managing medications, medical service, therapies or counseling, and other.

The most striking finding was the extreme rarity of any of these services being mentioned as unavailable by recent and longer-stay residents in either type of CCRC—so much so that a statistical comparison of the responses of residents in the two types of facility on an item-by-item basis was statistically inappropriate.[6]

Summary Measure of Service Availability. We constructed a summary measure of complaints about service availability by counting the number of times each resident mentioned that a service had been unavailable. Fewer than 10 percent of the recent and approximately 10 percent of the longer-stay residents of both types of CCRC reported that one or more of the services had been unavailable, and for almost all of these only one or two services were mentioned. Recording each unavailable service as a complaint, the mean number of service complaints was 0.35 for the recent residents of extended CCRCs and 0.60 for their

6. Among both recent and longer-stay residents of extended CCRCs, 3 percent wanting therapy was the largest group unable to get a service when needed. Among residents of limited CCRCs, the largest group finding services unavailable was 6 percent of the recent and 7 percent of the longer-stay residents saying they were unable to obtain help with chores.

counterparts in limited CCRCs; for longer-stay residents, the mean number was 0.25 and 0.62, respectively, for those in extended and limited CCRCs. Despite the few complaints, the differences between residents in these two types of CCRC were significant, and findings were similar when length of stay was broken down even further (see Table 3.5 and Appendix B, Table B7).

However, the frequency distributions for these constructed variables revealed that the differences were the result of the responses of a relatively small number of people, particularly in the longer-stay samples. Of recent residents with two or more complaints, only five were extended CCRC residents (1.8 percent of the sample of 281), and thirteen (5.9 percent of 220) were residents of limited CCRCs. Of longer-stay residents with two or more complaints, only five (0.9 percent of the 549) were residents of extended CCRCs, but twenty-nine (5 percent of 579) were residents of limited CCRCs. The major finding here was that these CCRC residents found that services, when needed, were almost always available.

Attitudes about CCRC at Baseline and Follow-Up

Three of the four attitudes probed at both baseline and at follow-up were related to satisfaction with specific aspects of the CCRC and its management. An additional question concerned the respondent's overall feeling about the CCRC living arrangement.

Specific Aspects of Living at the CCRC. The three questions tapping specific aspects of the CCRC at baseline and follow-up and the potential response options were:

- Do you, as a resident, have the opportunity to influence management decisions that affect you? [(1) Yes, (2) No]
- Are you satisfied with the social and leisure activities of this facility? [(1) Yes, (2) No]
- How do you feel about the amount of money you pay each month to live here? [(1) A bargain, (2) Just about right, (3) Too much]

The majority of all four samples responded favorably to these questions both at baseline and again at follow-up—that is, they claimed that they had the opportunity to influence management, were satisfied with social and leisure activities, and felt that the monthly amount of money paid to live at the CCRC was either just about right or a bargain (Table 3.6). The samples consistently responded least favorably to the question about their opportunity to influence management decisions. Further-

Table 3.5 Distribution of complaint responses of recent and longer-stay residents, by type of CCRC

	Recent				Longer-stay			
	Extended CCRC		Limited CCRC		Extended CCRC		Limited CCRC	
Score	Freq.	%	Freq.	%	Freq.	%	Freq.	%
0	225	80.1	167	75.9	486	88.5	421	72.7
1	27	9.6	18	8.2	21	3.8	59	10.2
2	20	7.1	15	6.8	23	4.2	48	8.3
3	6	2.1	9	4.1	12	2.2	19	3.3
4	2	0.7	5	2.3	5	0.9	21	3.6
5	1	0.4	1	0.5	1	0.2	5	0.9
6	0	0.0	4	1.8	0	0.0	4	0.7
7	0	0.0	1	0.5	1	0.2	2	0.3
Totals	281	100.0	220	100.0	549	100.0	579	100.0
	Mean scores							
	0.35		0.60[a]		0.25		0.62[b]	

[a]Differences between scale scores of recent residents of extended and limited CCRCs were statistically significant at $p \le 0.05$.

[b]Differences between scale scores of longer-stay (one year or more) residents of extended and limited CCRCs were statistically significant at $p \le 0.001$.

more, except at baseline for the sample of recent residents of extended CCRCs, more than 20 percent in each sample at both baseline and at follow-up felt that the amount of money they paid each month was too much.

There were several within-sample changes from baseline to follow-up as well as differences between residents of extended and limited CCRCs which were revealed by analyses comparing residents of extended and limited facilities at baseline and follow-up (t-test) and within-sample change (paired t-test). For recent samples, a significant within-sample decline occurred in both groups regarding their opportunity to influence management decisions that affected them. However, there were no significant differences between residents of extended and limited CCRCs at either baseline or follow-up for any of these variables. Furthermore, the logistic regression for ordinal categories (using baseline response and background characteristics as covariates to control for

Table 3.6 Satisfaction with specific aspects of the CCRC of recent and longer-stay residents of extended and limited CCRCs

		Recent				Longer-stay			
		Extended CCRC (N = 281)		Limited CCRC (N = 220)		Extended CCRC (N = 549)		Limited CCRC (N = 579)	
Variable	Response	Baseline	Follow-up	Baseline	Follow-up	Baseline	Follow-up	Baseline	Follow-up
		%	%	%	%	%	%	%	%
Opportunity to influence management?	Yes	79.5	66.2	75.8	64.1	71.8	66.3	64.6	58.6
Satisfied with social/leisure activities?	Yes	93.2	93.9	95.7	91.7	95.4	95.4	93.9	94.7
Amount of money each month to live here?	A bargain	5.5	6.2	6.5	9.3	9.4	10.8	9.1	13.1
	Just about right	76.2	69.1	71.0	64.0	68.9	68.4	58.1	59.4
	Too much	18.3	24.7	22.4	26.6	21.7	20.7	32.8	27.5

Note. Baseline differences were significant between longer-stay residents of extended and limited CCRCs regarding opportunity to influence management (t-test, $p \le 0.01$) and amount of money each month to live here ($p \le 0.001$). Follow-up differences were significant (t-test, $p \le 0.001$) between longer-stay residents of extended and limited CCRCs regarding opportunity to influence management. Baseline to follow-up difference (paired t-test, $p \le 0.05$) were significant for recent residents of extended and limited CCRCs and for longer-stay residents of limited CCRCs regarding opportunity to influence management.

baseline differences between the samples) did not change these findings. We can conclude that recent residents of the two types of CCRC held very similar opinions at follow-up about these three aspects of their CCRC.

As we found for recent residents, there were no significant differences in satisfaction with social and leisure activities between baseline and follow-up for the longer-stay residents in both types of facility, nor were there significant differences between residents in the two types of community either at baseline or at follow-up. Controlling for baseline characteristics did not change the follow-up finding of no difference between these residents. Of the three areas probed, social/leisure activities was the area of most satisfaction; at follow-up, 95 percent of the longer-stay residents in each type of CCRC expressed satisfaction with these activities at their CCRC.

Like the recent residents of both types of CCRC, longer-stay residents of limited CCRCs also experienced a significant decline in the percentage believing they had an opportunity to influence management. In contrast, the responses of these same residents were considerably more favorable at follow-up than at baseline for satisfaction with the amount of money paid for the monthly fee (responding that it was either a bargain or just about right).

There was no significant change in any of these three variables for longer-stay residents of extended CCRCs (although, like their counterparts in limited CCRCs, fewer persons at follow-up thought they had an opportunity to influence management). But both at baseline and at follow-up, significantly more of the longer-stay residents of extended CCRCs said they had an opportunity to influence management decisions. In addition, at baseline, but not at follow-up, longer-stay residents in extended CCRCs were less likely than residents of limited CCRCs to say that the amount of money spent each month to live at the CCRC was too much. In this case, however, controlling for baseline characteristics eliminated the differences at follow-up for the opportunity-to-influence-management variable and sustained the finding of no difference between residents of the two types of CCRC in their opinions as to the amount of money paid monthly to live in their community.

In general, controlled analyses indicate that at follow-up residents of extended and limited CCRCs felt similar degrees of satisfaction on these specific aspects of their community. It appears that the differential satisfaction of residents of extended and limited CCRCs at that point in time could have resulted from the types of people living at the CCRC and how they felt about these aspects of the CCRC at baseline.

General Attitude toward Living at the CCRC. The similarities and differences in satisfaction with these specific aspects of the CCRC provide contextual information as well as insights for interpreting overall attitudes toward the CCRC living arrangement. We asked a final global question, at both baseline and follow-up: "In general how do you feel about living here now?" The alternative responses were:

1. Distinctly positive feelings.
2. Ambivalent/mixed feelings.
3. Distinctly negative feelings.

We compared residents of the two types of CCRC at both points in time and analyzed within-sample changes. We performed logistic regression for ordinal categories to estimate probable outcome (follow-up responses) when background characteristics and baseline attitude were controlled.

Analysis of the overall feelings about the CCRC should provide insights as to the importance of previously explored attitudes, regarding both the extent to which they were reflected in general feelings of satisfaction in samples and whether there were significant differences between samples. Table 3.7 presents the distributions of the responses of the recent and longer-stay residents.

Residents of both types of CCRC, regardless of their length of residence, had quite positive attitudes. Among recent residents, 88 percent of those in extended CCRCs and 85 percent of those in limited CCRCs felt distinctly positive at baseline; at follow-up the comparable figures were 84 and 75 percent.

For the longer-stay residents, those in extended CCRCs had significantly more positive feelings about living at the CCRC at both baseline (85 percent) and follow-up (88 percent) than did the residents of limited CCRCs (79 percent at baseline and 78 percent at follow-up). For residents of extended CCRCs there was a small but significant increase in positive feelings from baseline to follow-up, but there was no change from baseline to follow-up for those in limited CCRCs.

Differences between samples on how residents felt about the CCRC in general followed a pattern similar to that of other responses at both baseline and follow-up. There was no significant difference between the samples of recent residents at baseline — a finding possibly understandable because the residents had relatively short amounts of time for experience to lessen the generally highly positive feelings at the outset of their tenure at the CCRC. For each of the remaining comparisons (including follow-up for recent residents), however, the findings were consistently more favorable for residents of extended than for limited CCRCs. Fur-

Table 3.7 General feelings about living at the CCRC

	Recent				Longer-stay			
	Extended CCRC (N = 281)		Limited CCRC (N = 220)		Extended CCRC (N = 549)		Limited CCRC (N = 579)	
Response	Baseline	Follow-up	Baseline	Follow-up	Baseline	Follow-up	Baseline	Follow-up
	%	%	%	%	%	%	%	%
Distinctly positive	88.2	84.2	84.5	75.0	84.7	87.6	78.9	78.0
Ambivalent/mixed	11.1	14.0	15.5	20.9	13.7	11.3	18.0	18.7
Distinctly negative	0.7	1.8	0.0	4.1	1.6	1.1	3.1	3.3

Note. The baseline difference was significant (*t*-test, $p \leq 0.01$) between longer-stay residents of extended and limited CCRCS. Follow-up differences were significant between recent residents of extended and limited CCRCs (*t*-test, $p \leq 0.01$) and between longer-stay residents of these two types of CCRC (*t*-test $p \leq 0.001$). Baseline to follow-up differences were significant for recent residents of limited CCRCs (paired *t*-test, $p \leq 0.001$) and for longer-stay residents of extended CCRCs (paired *t*-test, $p \leq 0.05$).

thermore, analyses controlling for differences in baseline characteristics supported the conclusions regarding differential outcome: both recent and longer-stay residents of extended CCRCs were more favorable even after controlling for baseline differences (i.e., it is likely that they would have been more positive than their counterparts in limited CCRCs even if the samples had been more alike at baseline). Thus, we could not account for the follow-up difference in satisfaction by the identified differences in background characteristics or resident attitudes at baseline.

Other Quality-of-Life Outcome Variables

At baseline and at follow-up we asked sample members a series of identical questions about various aspects of quality of life other than participation in activities and satisfaction with their CCRC, for example, component items of the previously standardized attitude-toward-own-aging scale (Morris and Sherwood 1975), pain experienced, visiting patterns, unmet needs. As was true for many of the individual satisfaction variables, very large proportions of residents, regardless of type of CCRC, responded in the same way to many of these questions. For example, between 97 and 99 percent of three of the samples both at baseline and at follow-up ventured out of the house more than one day a week, and, in the remaining sample (longer-stay residents in limited CCRCs), the percentages were 94 and 96 percent at baseline and follow-up, respectively. Comparisons involving composite scores of related variables were therefore more meaningful.

The final section of this chapter focuses on descriptions and controlled comparisons of residents of extended and limited CCRCs on two scales. These were:

- the previously standardized attitude-toward-own-aging scale;
- a constructed scale consisting of counts of positive responses to a cluster of variables identified through factor analysis, labeled the quality-of-life scale.

As in the previous analyses of satisfaction with the CCRC, we compared residents of extended and limited CCRCs at both baseline and follow-up, with separate analyses for recent and longer-stay residents. Focusing in particular on outcome at follow-up, we also addressed within-sample change between baseline and follow-up, and we present findings from controlled analyses (using logistic regression for ordinal categories with covariates) which estimated what differences there would have been in outcome at follow-up had the samples been similar in baseline characteristics and measures.

Attitude toward Own Aging

The attitude-toward-own-aging scale is a six-point index (from o to 5) based on the following five questions, in which o represents the most positive score (no negative feelings about their own aging), and 5 represents the most negative score (all responses indicated a negative feeling):

- Do you feel things keep getting worse as you get older?
- Do you feel you have as much pep as you did last year?
- As you get older, are you less useful?
- Are you as happy now as when you were younger?
- As you get older, would you say things are worse, the same, or better?

The majority of persons in each sample had no more than two negative responses. The mean scores for recent residents of extended CCRCs was 1.69 at baseline and 1.41 at follow-up; for residents of limited CCRCs, it was 1.84 and 1.35, respectively. For longer-stay residents of extended facilities, the mean scores at baseline and at follow-up were 2.04 and 1.99; for residents of limited CCRCs, the scores were 2.04 and 2.03 (see Table 3.8).

Both at baseline and at follow-up, there were no significant differences in attitude toward own aging between the residents of extended and limited CCRCs for either the recent or longer-stay samples. However, statistical analyses comparing the within-sample change (using the paired t-test) revealed some interesting findings. Although there were no significant within-sample changes for the longer-stay residents of either extended or limited CCRCs, significant within-sample changes from baseline to follow-up did occur for recent residents of both types of CCRC. In each case, their attitudes toward their own aging *improved significantly* from baseline to follow-up.

It is of course possible that although the overall samples appeared to be similar on the attitude-toward-own-aging scale, differences in attitude actually existed when background characteristics and baseline attitudes were controlled. Focusing on attitudes at follow-up, the question to address then is whether there would have been differential outcome when the baseline score on the attitude-toward-own-aging scale and key background characteristics were taken into consideration.

For the longer-stay residents, the answer was no — the finding of no difference between residents in the two types of CCRC was sustained. The answer for recent residents, however, was yes — differential outcome appeared to have been likely after baseline score and key background

Table 3.8 Distribution of scores and means on attitude-toward-own-aging scale of recent and longer-stay residents of extended and limited CCRCs

| | Recent | | | | Longer-stay | | | |
| | Extended CCRC (N = 281) | | Limited CCRC (N = 220) | | Extended CCRC (N = 549) | | Limited CCRC (N = 579) | |
Score[a]	Baseline	Follow-up	Baseline	Follow-up	Baseline	Follow-up	Baseline	Follow-up
	%	%	%	%	%	%	%	%
0	22.2	32.4	19.7	32.4	15.4	20.4	17.8	22.0
1	29.8	27.0	28.0	25.9	25.9	22.7	24.6	22.2
2	22.5	21.2	24.3	22.2	23.7	21.2	20.9	19.8
3	12.7	9.4	11.0	10.6	17.4	16.9	16.4	13.3
4	8.0	6.1	9.2	6.0	10.6	11.3	12.6	13.5
5	4.7	4.0	7.8	2.8	7.0	7.4	7.7	9.3
Mean scores								
	1.69	1.41*	1.84	1.35*	2.04	1.99	2.04	2.03

Note. An asterisk indicates that the within-sample change from baseline to follow-up was significant at the $p \leq 0.05$ level.

[a] 0 = most positive . . . 5 = most negative.

characteristics were considered. The recent residents of extended CCRCs would probably have had an even more positive attitude toward their own aging than the recent residents of limited CCRCs.

Quality-of-Life Scale Findings

The quality-of-life scale is a seven-point index (from 0 to 6), in which 6 represents the most positive score, and 0 represents the most negative score. The score represents a count of the most positive response category for each of six variables identified in the factor analyses conducted separately for recent and longer-stay samples. The six variables in this constructed scale and the response considered favorable for each are shown in Table 3.9.

The mean score on this quality-of-life scale for recent residents of extended CCRCs was 4.23 at baseline and 4.28 at follow-up; for residents of limited CCRCs it was 4.10 at baseline and 4.01 at follow-up. For longer-stay residents of extended facilities, the scores at baseline and at follow-up were 4.13 and 4.05; for residents of limited CCRCs, the mean score at baseline was 3.94 and at follow-up, 3.78.

As measured by this scale, the quality of life deteriorated significantly for longer-stay residents of limited CCRCs. For the remaining three within-sample comparisons, the scores at baseline and at follow-up were not significantly different, indicative of a relatively steady-state quality of life between these two periods of time (see Table 3.10).

There were between-sample differences, however, at follow-up (but not at baseline) between recent residents of extended and limited CCRCs and between longer-stay residents of these two types of CCRC both at baseline and at follow-up. In each case, the quality-of-life scores were significantly higher for residents of extended CCRCs. At the same time, the distributions were basically very similar; the great bulk of the residents of the two types of CCRC scored very similarly.

Recall that the discriminant function analysis revealed functional health at baseline as discriminating between longer-stay but not recent residents of the two types of CCRC. Two functional health items are part of this scale: perceptions of health and pain experienced. One might expect that controlling for baseline characteristics would change the findings, particularly for longer-stay residents. In fact, the regression estimate eliminated the follow-up difference between the recent residents of extended and limited CCRCs, but it sustained the follow-up difference between the longer-stay residents in the two types of facility: longer-stay extended CCRC residents had higher quality-of-life scores at follow-up even when controlling for their baseline differences with longer-stay lim-

Table 3.9 Quality-of-life scale

Variable	Most favorable response
How would you rate your health?	Excellent
How would you describe your pain?	No pain
How much of the time does your health prevent you from doing things you would like to do?	Seldom to never
Do you usually go out of the house (building in which you live) more than one day a week?	Yes
During the past week, how much time did you spend chatting on the phone or visiting in person with your friends?	Considerable
Unmet needs index[a]	No unmet needs (in seven ADL/IADL areas)

[a]At both the baseline and follow-up interviews, we asked sample members whether it would have been helpful if they had personally received (more) assistance for the following ADL/IADL areas: light housekeeping, chores, shopping, meals, personal care, medications, and transporation. As occurred regarding availability of services, the distribution of responses in each of these areas was very skewed, with very few persons reporting the need for more assistance. The composite scale score for this cluster of variables was considered more meaningful.

ited CCRC residents.[7] There did appear to be a difference in the quality of life between the two longer-stay groups at follow-up, at least as measured by responses to these six questions, and this difference could not be explained by differences at baseline or differences with respect to the fifteen covariates utilized in the analysis.

Conclusions and Insights

Overall, the findings for each of the analyses revealed a remarkable similarity in the pattern of responses across all four samples. This included the use of CCRC amenities, participation in activities both before and after joining the CCRC, attitudes and perceptions of the CCRC living arrangement, and scores on other selected quality-of-life indices. However, there were significant differences (often small) between residents in the two types of facility, and when they were found, they were generally in favor of the residents of extended CCRCs. Such findings have implications for CCRC developers and operators as well as for elderly persons who are planning their future and are considering joining a CCRC.

7. Because the distribution of responses to this set of questions was approximately normal, we also performed an analysis of covariance; it produced the same finding.

Table 3.10 Distribution of scores and means on quality-of-life scale of recent and longer-stay residents of extended and limited CCRCs

	Recent				Longer-stay			
	Extended CCRC (N = 281)		Limited CCRC (N = 220)		Extended CCRC (N = 549)		Limited CCRC (N = 579)	
Score[a]	Baseline	Follow-up	Baseline	Follow-up	Baseline	Follow-up	Baseline	Follow-up
	%	%	%	%	%	%	%	%
0	0.4	0.0	0.0	0.5	0.2	0.2	0.9	0.2
1	1.1	2.5	1.4	0.0	1.5	1.2	2.2	1.9
2	5.0	5.0	5.0	5.0	4.7	6.9	8.8	12.2
3	16.4	10.7	17.7	23.2	19.1	18.9	16.4	21.9
4	34.9	35.6	40.5	40.5	36.1	38.1	39.4	38.9
5	30.2	35.9	28.6	25.9	30.2	26.2	26.1	20.0
6	12.1	10.3	6.8	5.0	8.2	8.2	6.2	5.0
Mean scores								
	4.23	4.28	4.10	4.01	4.13	4.05	3.94	3.78*

Note. Asterisk indicates that the within-sample change from baseline to follow-up was significant at the $p \leq 0.05$ level.

[a] 6 = most positive . . . 0 = most negative.

Activities

The pattern of use of CCRC amenities available in all nineteen communities was identical across all four groups with regard to rank order of percentages of users: library, chapel, crafts/activities room, game room, and health club/exercise classes. As many as 80 percent or more of the recent and longer-stay residents of extended CCRCs used the library, but only about 20 percent used the health club or attended exercise classes. Among recent and longer-stay residents of limited CCRCs, 66 and 78 percent, respectively, used the library, but only 26 and 20 percent, respectively, used the health club or attended exercise classes. In general, differences in the extended and limited CCRC residents' use of CCRC amenities appeared to be a function of differences in the characteristics (health, age, and related variables) of the samples of residents rather than characteristics of the facilities.

There was considerable similarity across samples, regardless of length of residence, in the pattern of participation in activities while a CCRC resident. CCRC residents appear to be an active population, generally participating in half or more of the fifteen activities probed (and probably participating in other activities that were not queried). On the whole, the extended CCRC residents participated in significantly more activities than did the residents of limited CCRCs and were more likely to participate in some activities (e.g., lectures), but residents of limited CCRCs were more likely to participate in volunteer activities. Furthermore, although health and age were related to participation, differences in age and health did not account for the differences observed between residents of the two types of CCRC.

All groups engaged in fewer activities than they had as younger adults (before joining the CCRC), and only a small percentage in any of the groups participated in new types of activity after joining the CCRC. Although no more than 7 percent did so in any of the samples, attending lectures and volunteer activities elicited the highest percentage of new participants. Approximately 4 percent of the recent residents in both types of CCRC attended lectures.

Residents' Attitudes and Perceptions of the
CCRC Living Arrangement

In general, residents in both types of facility tended to be very satisfied with the CCRC. A large majority of all groups were satisfied with housing and with the cost of living at the CCRC, thought they had made a good decision in moving there, and would have recommended the

CCRC to others. Ninety-five percent or more thought that it had been a good decision to move to the CCRC. Residents of extended CCRCs were particularly positive. For example, 96 percent of the recent residents and 99 percent of those of longer stay thought it had been a good decision to move to the CCRC; 98 percent of the recent and 96 percent of the longer-stay residents would have recommended the CCRC to others. Furthermore, according to the general satisfaction summary measure (constructed for the six questions pertaining to satisfaction asked at follow-up only), the average number of favorable responses was significantly higher for residents of extended than for residents of limited CCRCs.

Although less so for residents of extended CCRCs, sizable minorities said that the CCRC did not meet their expectations — as many as 22 and 39 percent, respectively, of the recent residents of extended and limited CCRCs, and 13 and 30 percent, respectively, of the longer-stay residents of extended and limited CCRCs. This suggests that at least some persons entering these communities have unrealistic ideas of what to expect. This finding should give CCRC operators and developers and those marketing them food for thought.

The relatively high percentages of each group voicing no opinion about the care given at the CCRC nursing home (health center) and the stark difference between residents of extended and limited CCRCs in this regard are also noteworthy. Of recent residents, 28 percent of the extended and as many as 46 percent of those in limited CCRCs said they had no opinion; of the longer-stay residents, the corresponding percentages were 19 and 32. The differences between residents of extended and limited CCRCs are, perhaps, not surprising in view of the significantly larger proportions of residents of extended than of limited CCRCs who considered availability of the nursing home important in their choice of CCRC. One might expect that residents who are concerned about the issue of potential need for nursing home care would take an interest (and thus have an opinion) in the quality of care provided in the health center. The smaller proportions with no opinion on this issue among the longer-stay residents are also not surprising. The more the opportunity for experience with the care provided (either personal experience or through visiting friends at the health center) and/or the greater the relevance to the resident (e.g., interest with advancing age and deteriorating health status), the more likely the residents will learn about and have an opinion on the care provided.

Of those who expressed an opinion, close to 90 percent or more of the recent residents in both types of facility were satisfied with the care given at the health center. Of the longer-stay residents, there was a similar percentage for extended CCRC residents, although still a large majority, but significantly fewer residents of limited CCRCs (82 percent) were satisfied with the care provided at the health center.

Undoubtedly related to the high degree of satisfaction of all groups, a striking finding was the extreme rarity of persons who said that they had ever experienced a time when they were unable to get services when needed. For almost all persons who reported that there was a time when one or more (of the ten) services were unavailable when needed, only one or two services were mentioned.

Table 3.11 summarizes the responses to the four baseline and follow-up questions that directly or indirectly pertained to satisfaction with the CCRC. Responses pertaining to specific aspects of the CCRC probed at baseline and follow-up were consistent with previous findings regarding questions about satisfaction which we asked only at follow-up. The majority of all four groups said they had the opportunity to influence management decisions that affected them, were satisfied with the CCRC social and leisure activities, and felt that the amount of money spent each month to live at the facility was either just about right or a bargain.

Nevertheless, sizable minorities (ranging from approximately 20 to 40 percent) of each of the samples responded unfavorably to the questions about influencing management and monthly payments both at baseline and at follow-up. By follow-up, between 34 percent (recent and longer-stay extended CCRC residents) and 41 percent (longer-stay limited CCRC residents) said they did not have the opportunity to influence management decisions that affected them, and between 21 percent (longer-stay extended CCRC residents) and 28 percent (longer-stay limited CCRC residents) felt that the amount of money was too much. If we can presume that the monthly charges were actually reasonable, given inflation and actual expenses, this suggests that CCRCs should be thinking about strategies by which residents could understand better the basis for determining the monthly fees and/or why they need to be as high as they are. CCRCs might, for example, consider involving the residents more in this process. By doing so, more of the CCRC residents might feel that they, indeed, had an opportunity to influence management.

Although recent residents in both types of CCRC responded similarly to these questions, longer-stay residents of extended CCRCs were more likely to respond favorably to them both at baseline and follow-up. Differences regarding satisfaction with the amount of money paid each month to live at the facility were in line with responses to the question about whether the cost of living at the CCRC was a good value (asked at follow-up only), with longer-stay residents of limited CCRCs responding less favorably than their counterparts in extended CCRCs. These differ-

Table 3.11 Satisfaction variables probed at baseline and at follow-up

Recent residents

Variable	Change baseline to post-test		Comparison extended vs. limited		Follow-up scores estimated by logistic regression
	Extended	Limited	Baseline	Follow-up	
Opportunity to influence management	Negative	Negative	No difference	No difference	No difference
Satisfied with the social and leisure activities	None	None	No difference	No difference	No difference
Feel about amount of money paid monthly to live at CCRC	None	None	No difference	No difference	No difference
Feelings about living in CCRC in general	None	Negative	No difference	Extended more positive	Extended more favorable

Longer-stay residents

Variable	Change baseline to post-test		Comparison extended vs. limited		Follow-up scores estimated by logistic regression
	Extended	Limited	Baseline	Follow-up	
Opportunity to influence management	None	Negative	Extended more positive	Extended more positive	No difference
Satisfied with the social and leisure activities	None	None	No difference	No difference	No difference
Feel about amount of money paid monthly to live at CCRC	None	Positive	Extended more positive	Extended more positive	No difference
Feelings about living in CCRC in general	Positive	No difference	Extended more positive	Extended more positive	Extended more favorable

ences between longer-stay residents in the two types of CCRC are interesting in the light of differences in the average monthly fees of these two types of CCRC as well as the previous difference in responses to a question asked at baseline regarding satisfaction with the entry fee. Using the monthly fees in place at their CCRC at the time of the baseline interview as the foundation for analysis, the average monthly fee was significantly higher for residents of extended CCRCs than for those of limited CCRCs ($965 and $674, respectively). Longer-stay limited CCRC sample members nevertheless expressed greater dissatisfaction with the amount of money paid each month.

We found differential satisfaction at follow-up between residents of the two types of CCRC regarding cost and the opportunity to influence management. These differences could have been the result of the types of individuals living at the CCRCs and how they felt about these aspects of the CCRC at baseline. But baseline differences between the residents of extended and limited CCRCs do not explain the follow-up differences between the longer-stay samples on how they felt about the CCRC in general. Although responses tended to be positive for residents of both types of CCRC regardless of the length of residence, at follow-up the responses of recent and longer-stay residents of extended CCRCs were more favorable than those of their counterparts in limited CCRCs. These differences could not be explained by the identified differences in background characteristics or their attitudes at baseline. In other words, for persons with similar characteristics at baseline, it is reasonable to conclude that there was differential outcome at follow-up in favor of the residents of extended CCRCs.

Considering the entire set of questions either directly or indirectly reflecting satisfaction with the CCRC, including those that we asked only at follow-up and those that we asked both at baseline and follow-up, a fair conclusion is that residents of extended CCRCs were more satisfied in general about their CCRC than were residents of limited CCRCs. We should reemphasize, however, that both recent and longer-stay residents of both types of CCRC appeared to be very satisfied with their CCRC.

Other Quality-of-Life Outcomes

Findings from the analyses of other quality-of-life variables rounded out this picture. The patterns of responses of all four samples were very similar on both of these indices. However, longer-stay residents of extended CCRCs appeared to do better than their counterparts in limited CCRCs regarding quality of life as measured by the constructed quality-of-life scale. Analyses controlling for initial differences in the two populations supported these findings.

Finally, the findings pertaining to the attitude-toward-own-aging scale yielded some interesting insights. No differences were found between longer-stay residents of the two types of CCRC, nor were there significant within-sample changes for these residents. But there were significant within-sample changes from baseline to follow-up for recent residents of both types of CCRC. Although the controlled analysis indicated that the recent residents of extended CCRCs would have had even more positive attitudes had the two samples been more alike, both in limited and extended CCRCs the residents' attitudes toward their own aging improved significantly from baseline to follow-up. This suggests that CCRCs, regardless of type, provide a different type of environment than is likely to be found in traditional-community living arrangements. The CCRCs furnish an environment conducive to positive adaptation of the picture residents have of their own aging. Further, it does not take long for such positive adaptation to occur, and this process may be even stronger in extended CCRC environments. However, to the extent that the longer-stay residents represent the recent residents at a later point in their lives, it appears that attitudes toward their own aging do not continue to improve but rather tend to level off at a somewhat more negative level. After a number of years at the CCRC, it is reasonable to suppose that the residents' reference group for their own aging is no longer their traditional-community peers but rather peers within the CCRC itself. Although their morale may slacken somewhat as they grow older, this would seem to be a slow process, certainly not reflected by a significant change between baseline and follow-up measures a year to a year and one-half apart.

FOUR

Quality of Life in CCRC
and Community Elderly Populations

In Chapter 1, we compared recent and longer-stay CCRC residents who were at least 70 years old with their age peers in the Massachusetts community on demographic characteristics and quality-of-life descriptors such as health, functional status, social interaction, and informal supports. In this chapter we report our analyses of the changes in such characteristics for sample members who were alive and had follow-up interviews approximately sixteen months after the baseline interview, and we compare the CCRC residents (combining the subsamples of recent and longer-stay residents of extended and limited CCRCs) with their counterparts in the Massachusetts community.

We analyzed these two samples at two points in time and assessed the outcome at follow-up. It is important to stress that from these analyses we can make no determination of the impact of CCRCs as opposed to that of traditional-community living arrangements. This study did not employ an experimental design in which eligible applicants to CCRCs were randomly offered residence and others were not. Nor did we employ a quasi-experimental design. CCRC sample members all sought out a CCRC and made the decision to enter on their own. Furthermore, no baseline data before the move to the CCRC were available, nor did we gather comparable data for a sample of eligible elderly persons known to be interested or potentially interested in this type of living arrangement but who did not enter a CCRC.

CCRCs are designed, at least to some extent, as pooled-risk living arrangements that allow aging in place. At one extreme, they provide independent living in one's own apartment and, when needed, long-term nursing care, generally in the same location. Elderly traditional-community residents live in many types of housing (e.g., private home, age-integrated apartment buildings, age-segregated public housing) and in different types of living arrangements, both regarding head of household (living in their own apartment or house or in the home of others) and with whom they live (alone or, in various combinations, with others — spouse, children, grandchildren). In short, despite some diversity among

CCRCs, compared with the heterogeneity of the traditional community, almost all CCRC residents lived alone or with a spouse in relatively similar (to other CCRC residents) situations.

Although the market is expanding, to date only a small proportion of elderly persons have joined CCRCs, and persons who become residents of this type of community are not representative of elderly persons in general. Evidence from this and other studies reveals consistently that CCRC residents are drawn from the older segments of the elderly population, the age groups in which the specter of future medical problems and decreased functioning is likely to be a more immediate reality. CCRCs appear to attract persons whose life style is to plan ahead and not be dependent upon family or friends either to provide the bulk of supportive services or to make decisions for them. CCRCs also appeal to elderly persons without children or other family members on whom they could rely if they were to become sick and require long-term help.

However, a CCRC might not be economically feasible for many persons who would otherwise find them attractive. Although most CCRCs at the present time are nonprofit, they are private enterprises that require considerable up-front money as an entrance fee as well as monthly fees that are sufficiently large to cover not only housing and amenities but also, whether on a completely or very limited pooled-risk basis, future potential costs of nursing home care. For all practical purposes, personal financial solvency and stability are eligibility requirements for residence in this type of community.

Furthermore, entrants to an apartment in a CCRC must generally be in sufficiently good health and physical functioning so as not to need extensive supportive services or to be likely prospects for nursing home placement in the immediate or near future. Some CCRCs specify preexisting medical problems for which the CCRC will not be financially responsible. Thus, CCRCs are likely to draw upon the segments of the elderly population which are healthier, at least for their age group.

In addition to key selection biases, it is also possible that the CCRC way of life has an impact on quality-of-life outcomes (e.g., health, functional status, and social interactions). Thus, at baseline, we expected (and demonstrated empirically by the analyses in Chapter 1) that there are major differences between the CCRC and traditional-community populations.

The primary focus in this chapter, then, is on a comparison of the follow-up outcome variables of CCRC residents and those of elderly traditional-community residents, as represented by the Massachusetts sample. We considered baseline differences between these two samples primarily to assess changes that occurred from baseline to follow-up, both in univariate analyses and as covariates in more controlled comparisons. In particular, we address the following questions:

- How different are these samples from each other on these quality-of-life outcome variables at baseline and at a comparable follow-up point? Do baseline differences persist? Do new differences appear?
- How do these two samples — CCRC residents and traditional-community residents 70 years of age and older — change over time? For each key quality-of-life outcome variable for which comparable baseline and follow-up data are available, is the nature of the change similar or different for the two samples?
- For each outcome variable, how would CCRC residents have fared at follow-up compared with traditional-community residents when selection biases predictive of group membership, their baseline scores, and time between baseline and follow-up are considered?

Samples, Data Sources, and Analyses

CCRCs attract the older segments of the elderly population, and very few of the CCRC sample members in this study were younger than 70 years. To make the analyses more meaningful, we restricted comparisons with traditional-community residents to persons who were at least 70 years old. The findings, then, pertain to comparisons between the combined sample of CCRC residents of this age group and the overall representative sample of their Massachusetts age peers.

We derived data about the CCRC residents from the baseline interviews we conducted during 1986 and early 1987 as well as the follow-up interviews. Comparable data for elderly traditional-community residents came from the interviews conducted in the Massachusetts study during approximately the same periods of time (hereinafter also referred to as baseline and follow-up), but, on average, the time period between baseline and follow-up was approximately eighteen months, a little longer than in the CCRC study.

Samples

CCRC sample members in these comparisons were people living in apartments at baseline, alive at follow-up, and for whom follow-up data were available. The comparison sample consisted of Massachusetts community residents at baseline who were alive at follow-up and for whom follow-up interviews were available.[1]

---

1. For the few persons who were alive at follow-up but who could not be interviewed, we obtained information regarding their functional status and behavior from a significant

We could not obtain usable follow-up interviews for some of the baseline sample because the person had died, moved out of the area permanently, refused to be interviewed, or was not accessible.[2] Of the overall baseline samples, follow-up information pertinent to the analyses presented in this chapter was available for 1,576 (or 80 percent) of the overall sample of 1,970 CCRC residents who were at least 70 years old at baseline and 1,266 (or 89 percent) of the overall baseline sample of 1,430 Massachusetts age peers.

Outcome Variables

Outcome variables available for analysis were only those for which we obtained comparable measures at baseline and follow-up for both samples. The variables we considered components of the quality of life were: health (three variables), physical and mental functioning (five variables), social interaction and informal supports (six variables), and others such as inner resources and unmet needs (three variables).

Analyses

We performed simple chi-squares and *t*-tests comparing separately the baseline and follow-up differences between the CCRC and Massachusetts cohorts. We used paired *t*-tests in the intrasample comparisons of change from baseline to follow-up. For the remaining analyses we employed multivariate techniques. To identify key biases predictive of group membership we performed discriminant function analysis. We used logistic regression for ordinal categories (with covariates) to adjust for these selection biases, the initial difference on the baseline measure of the outcome variable, and the difference in time between baseline and follow-up. These controlled analyses, therefore, provided an estimate regarding probable outcome, assuming that the time between baseline and follow-up was the same and that the two samples were more alike on the identified key baseline characteristics (reducing the possibility that

---

other in the best position to answer the questions (e.g., spouse, child or other relative, friend). By comparing proxy information with data derived only from interviews with the elderly persons themselves we determined that inclusion of proxy data did not distort our conclusions. Therefore, our findings here include information gained from both types of source.

2. Of the total baseline sample of CCRC residents 6.4 percent had died. For 13.2 percent we obtained only limited information not pertinent to the quality-of-life analyses. In a few cases (0.4 percent), some of the residents had moved out of the CCRC between baseline and follow-up, and we were unable to obtain their follow-up address. Of the Massachusetts baseline sample 7.3 percent had died, and for the remaining 4.1 percent we obtained only limited information not pertinent to the quality-of-life analyses.

observed differences could result from differences in characteristics of the two samples or the differences in the time between baseline and follow-up rather than the environment/living arrangement).

Discriminant Function Analysis

The discriminant function analysis utilized demographic and other variables available in both the CCRC and Massachusetts baseline data sets representing conceptually relevant domains: age, sex, economic and educational status, marital status, availability of close family on whom to depend, independence in decision making, health, and functional status. Of these, nine baseline variables were identified. Seven were demographic characteristics: age, sex, education, income, living alone/not alone, number (up to eight) of children nearby (within a one-hour drive), and whether a spouse was part of the informal support system (i.e., when the resident was sick and required help, the spouse provided/could be relied upon to provide help). Two were health/functional status variables: number of limiting health/medical problems and the ability to do one's own shopping or perform small errands. In combination, even after the discriminant function analysis considered intercorrelations and eliminated shared contributions of these variables to the prediction equation, each variable made a significant independent contribution to the prediction of group membership. Table 4.1 presents the variables, the baseline mean scores and standard deviations for each group, as well as the standardized canonical discriminant function coefficient for each of these nine variables. They are ordered by canonical coefficient size, from highest to lowest, indicative of the importance of the variable in contributing to the prediction of group membership.

The discriminant function equation predicted correct sample membership 86 percent of the time: 87 percent of the CCRC sample members and 85 percent of the Massachusetts residents. This prediction rate indicates that our list of covariates accounted for many of the structural factors that differentiated the two samples. We then considered these nine variables basic and used them as covariates in each of the logistic regressions for ordinal categories (the adjusted outcome analyses). Thus, we statistically controlled the intersample differences for these factors, within the limitations of the correlations of these variables with the dependent variables.

The variable with the highest discriminant coefficient was age, a generally recognized major biasing characteristic of CCRC residents which differentiates them from elderly traditional-community residents. The CCRC residents had a higher mean age at baseline (approximately 81 years nine months) than the Massachusetts population (with a mean

Table 4.1 Baseline variables identified by the discriminant function equation predicting group membership, CCRC or Massachusetts elderly, ordered by size of standardized canonical discriminant function coefficient

Variable	CCRC		MA elderly		Standardized discriminant function canonical correlation coefficient
	Mean	S.D.	Mean	S.D.	
Age in years	81.73	5.60	77.59	5.80	0.55101
Income	2.67	1.37	1.52	0.85	0.47890
1 = up to $20,000					
2 = $20,001–$30,000					
3 = $30,001–$40,000					
4 = $40,001–$50,000					
5 = over $50,000					
Years of education	14.75	3.04	10.99	3.35	0.47165
Able to shop/do small errands	0.29	0.78	0.75	1.16	−0.40698
[0 = without help . . .					
4 = can't do at all]					
Sex [1 = male; 2 = female]	1.76	0.43	1.60	0.49	0.34527
No. of children nearby	0.37	0.67	1.34	1.46	−0.31986
[0 = none . . . 8 = 8 or more]					
No. of limiting medical problems	0.75	1.07	0.63	1.02	0.24174
(of 10) [0 = 0 . . . 10 = 10]					
Spouse is a helper	0.36	0.48	0.40	0.49	0.22685
[1 = yes; 0 = no]					
Lives alone [1 = yes; 0 = no]	0.59	0.49	0.43	0.50	0.19883

age of approximately 77 years seven months). Almost one third of the CCRC residents (31 percent) compared with 13 percent of the Massachusetts sample was at least 85 years old at baseline.

Income and education had the next highest discriminant coefficients, followed by the extent to which the sample member could shop or perform small errands. Each of these variables made a strong independent contribution to the prediction of group membership. As a group, the CCRC residents were wealthier and better educated than the Massachusetts sample. More than half of the CCRC sample (52 percent) had graduated from college, and only 23 percent had an income of no more than $20,000. In contrast, only 10 percent of the Massachusetts sample had graduated from college, and as many as two thirds had an income of no more than $20,000. Despite their older age, the CCRC residents also tended to be more independent than the Massachusetts group in shopping and performing small errands. As many as 85 percent of the CCRC residents compared with 65 percent of the Massachusetts group could perform these tasks completely on their own; less than 10 percent of the CCRC population but more than one quarter of the Massachusetts sample needed help most or all of the time in shopping and performing small errands.

The three variables next in order which contributed independently to the discriminant function equation were sex, number of children nearby, and number of limiting medical problems. A larger proportion of the CCRC population was female, more than three quarters of the CCRC residents compared with 60 percent of the Massachusetts sample. Proportionately many more CCRC residents (72 percent) than elderly Massachusetts residents (26 percent) had no children living within a one-hour drive.

For both samples, the average number of limiting medical problems was less than one.[3] But CCRC residents tended to have a greater number of limiting medical problems than did the Massachusetts group. Thirty-seven percent of the Massachusetts sample compared with 43 percent of the CCRC sample had one or more limiting medical problems.

Slightly more of the Massachusetts sample (40 percent) than of the CCRC sample (36 percent) had a spouse who either provided help or could be relied upon if help were needed. Similarly, CCRC residents age 70 and older were more likely to live alone than their age peers in the Massachusetts community (59.1 and 43.1 percent, respectively).

Quality-of-Life Outcomes

We have summarized quality-of-life findings separately for each of the following: perceived health, functional status, social interaction and informal supports, and inner resources and unmet needs. See Appendix B, Table B8, for details concerning the scoring of the variables and the mean scores at baseline and follow-up of the samples of CCRC and traditional-community residents.

Perceived Health Status

The perceived health domain consisted of three measures: self-reported rating of general health; pain rating; and perception of the extent to which bad health, sickness, or pain had prevented the respondent from doing things she or he would like to have done. Table 4.2 summa-

---

3. Many more, in fact the large majority, in both samples had one or more of the ten medical problems probed (91 percent in the CCRC and 84 percent in the Massachusetts samples), but often the respondents did not consider such conditions limiting.

Table 4.2 Perceived health

Variable	Comparison of CCRC vs. MA		Change from baseline to follow-up		Follow-up scores estimated by logistic regression[a]
	Baseline	Follow-up	CCRC sample	MA sample	
Self-reported rating of general health	CCRC better health	CCRC better health	Poorer health	Poorer health	No difference
Pain rating	CCRC less pain	CCRC less pain	More pain	More pain	No difference
Sickness or pain prevents doing what one wants	CCRC prevented less	CCRC prevented less	Prevented more	Prevented more	No difference

[a]Logistic regression for ordinal categories.

rizes the results of the *t*-test, the paired *t*-test, and logistic regression for each variable. The direction of significant differences, if any, resulted from comparisons between CCRC and Massachusetts traditional-community residents at baseline and at follow-up (the *t*-test); the direction of the change, if it occurred, from baseline to follow-up within each sample (the paired *t*-test); and, if an estimated follow-up difference between the CCRC and Massachusetts samples was predicted when key biases were controlled (the logistic regression comparisons), the direction of the difference (the results of the logistic regression procedures).

Both the CCRC and Massachusetts traditional-community residents were significantly worse off at follow-up than at baseline. Nevertheless, in both groups, a large percentage indicated at follow-up that they were either in good or excellent health (75 percent of the CCRC residents and 67 percent of the Massachusetts sample). The majority at follow-up also indicated that they did not experience any pain (62 percent of the CCRC residents and 64 percent of the Massachusetts sample). Furthermore, although health more frequently prevented desired activities at follow-up than at baseline for persons in both populations, at follow-up only 16 percent of the CCRC sample and 20 percent of the Massachusetts sample said that bad health, sickness, or pain had frequently stopped them from doing things they would like to have done.

Notwithstanding the younger average age of the Massachusetts sample, we observed differences at baseline and at follow-up in favor of the CCRC sample for all three perceived health variables. Even though they had a greater number of limiting medical problems, the CCRC residents perceived themselves to have been in better health, to have experienced less pain, and to have been less frequently prevented from doing what they wanted. However, findings from the controlled analyses (logistic regressions) indicated no differences between CCRC and Massachusetts residents at follow-up for any of the perceived health variables. It appears that differences in baseline characteristics accounted for the unadjusted follow-up differences.

Functional Status (Mental and Physical)

Five mental and functional status variables were investigated:

- orientation to time and place (mental status);
- a constructed scale measuring level of self-sufficiency;
- a constructed scale measuring ability to perform basic activities of daily living (ADL index): dressing, bathing, personal care, managing medications, and getting out of a chair;
- a constructed mobility impairment index, measuring the use of a

walker/wheelchair, climbing stairs, ability to walk (or wheel) twenty feet or a half-mile;

- a constructed scale measuring the ability to perform instrumental tasks of daily living (IADL index): taking out garbage, doing light housekeeping, chores, preparing meals, going shopping and running small errands, using transportation.

Table 4.3 summarizes the findings for each of these variables.

Although very large majorities in both samples attained a perfect score at follow-up on the mental status scale (94 percent of the CCRC sample and 96 percent of the Massachusetts sample), some deterioration in mental status from baseline to follow-up had occurred in both groups. There was no difference between the CCRC and Massachusetts samples in mental status either at baseline and follow-up, and the similarity in outcome for these two populations was sustained even after adjusting for baseline characteristics.

At baseline and at follow-up, the Massachusetts group scored more poorly than the CCRC residents on all four of the physical functional status variables, and both samples experienced significant deterioration in all four areas. However, we should emphasize that for many of the components of these scales, 80 percent or more of each sample at follow-up gave the most positive response. For example, 91 percent of each sample was independent in dressing; 86 percent of the CCRC residents and 84 percent of the Massachusetts elders were healthy enough to walk up and down stairs without help. In fact, although the CCRC residents were somewhat more likely to be independent in ADLs, the difference between the samples was small (92 vs. 91 percent at baseline and 86 vs. 84 percent at follow-up), and it reflected mostly a difference in bathing (where 11 percent of Massachusetts group and 7 percent of CCRC residents required help at baseline), the first area in which self-sufficiency tends to deteriorate. For later ADL losses, such as transfer (getting out of a chair without help), there was no difference in dependence rates.

After controlling for key baseline differences and the time between baseline and follow-up, only one difference remained: according to the estimates from the logistic regression analysis, CCRC residents had fewer IADL problems than did Massachusetts residents. Although the Massachusetts residents were less likely to be independent in IADLs at baseline (43 vs. 55 percent for CCRC residents) and at follow-up (37 vs. 43 percent), the difference at follow-up in favor of the CCRC residents could result in part from a sharper decline in the percentage of the Massachusetts group still able to do chores without help (e.g. washing floors, hanging curtains, defrosting the refrigerator, moving furniture). The per-

Table 4.3 Functional and mental status

| Variable | Comparison of CCRC vs. MA | | Change from baseline to follow-up | | Follow-up scores estimated by logistic regression[a] |
	Baseline	Follow-up	CCRC sample	MA sample	
Self-sufficiency	CCRC more self-sufficient	CCRC more self-sufficient	Less self-sufficient	Less self-sufficient	No difference
ADL index	CCRC fewer impairments	CCRC fewer impairments	More impairments	More impairments	No difference
Mobility index	CCRC more mobile	CCRC more mobile	Less mobile	Less mobile	No difference
IADL	CCRC had fewer problems	CCRC had fewer problems	More problems	More problems	CCRC would have had fewer problems
Mental status	No difference	No difference	More impairments	More impairments	No difference

[a]Logistic regression for ordinal categories.

centage of elderly Massachusetts residents who were independent dropped from 48 percent at baseline to 32 percent at follow-up and from 32 to 23 percent for the CCRC residents. The CCRC environment affords fewer opportunities to perform chores than does a community residence, particularly when that residence is a house rather than an apartment. It may be that elderly residents of the traditional community have a better basis for assessing their abilities in this area. At the same time, with meals, light housekeeping, and the chore services received, the CCRC residents may have more residual energy to perform chores when necessary. Their ability to meet societal and environmental demands in performing these and other IADLs thus may very well be less affected by deteriorating health status and deteriorating basic ADL capacities.

Social Interaction and Informal Supports

The activities/social interaction domain consisted of four measures: going out of the house (building in which the resident lived) more than once a week; time spent phoning or visiting friends; time spent phoning or visiting relatives; and the presence or absence of a confidante, that is, someone to whom they felt particularly close, with whom they could be completely themselves, and in whom they had total trust and confidence. The informal support domain contained two measures: the number of people who provided help or who would have provided help if needed and the number who could be relied upon to provide care indefinitely or for as long as needed. Table 4.4 describes the results of the t-test, the paired t-test, and logistic regression.

At both baseline and follow-up, CCRC residents were more likely than the Massachusetts residents to venture out of their houses or buildings more than once a week. The large majority of both populations, however, continued to do so more than once a week at follow-up. Nonetheless, significantly fewer of the Massachusetts sample went out (91 percent at baseline compared with 86 percent at follow-up). No drop in this activity occurred for the CCRC sample (96 percent went out more than once a week at baseline and 97 percent at follow-up). Even after controlling for key baseline differences between the samples and time between baseline and follow-up, the difference in favor of CCRC residents remained.

To the extent that this finding reflected some real differences between the two samples, it probably results from a combination of CCRC environmental factors (compared with those in which many of the Massachusetts sample members live), including the fact that most CCRCs have a number of leisure resources and activity programs either on-site

Table 4.4 Social interaction and informal supports

Variable	Comparison of CCRC vs. MA		Change from baseline to follow-up		Follow-up scores estimated by logistic regression[a]
	Baseline	Follow-up	CCRC sample	MA sample	
Goes out of house more than once a week	CCRC go out more	CCRC go out more	No change	Go out less	CCRC residents would go out more
Time spent phoning or visiting friends	CCRC residents spent more time	CCRC residents spent more time	Spent more time	No change	CCRC residents would spend more time
Time spent phoning or visting family	MA elderly spent more time	MA elderly spent more time	Spent more time	Spent more time	MA elderly would spend more time
Whether respondent has a confidante	More MA elderly had a confidante	More MA elderly had a confidante	No change	No change	More MA elderly would have a confidante
No. of informal helpers who could provide help if needed	No difference	MA elderly had more helpers	Fewer helpers	More helpers	MA elderly would have more helpers
No. of informal helpers who could be relied upon for as long as needed	MA elderly had more helpers	No difference	Fewer helpers	Fewer helpers	CCRC residents would have more helpers

[a]Logistic regression for ordinal categories.

or with transportation provided. Massachusetts sample members generally do not live in such circumstances.

The CCRC residents significantly increased the time spent phoning and visiting friends during the baseline to follow-up study period; 36 percent spent considerable time in this type of interaction at baseline and 47 percent at follow-up. The Massachusetts residents spent approximately the same time interacting by phone or visits with friends (39 percent at baseline and 40 percent at follow-up). At both points in time, CCRC residents were likely to spend significantly more time than Massachusetts residents in such activities, and the logistic regression procedure estimated that the difference in outcome at follow-up would remain even after controlling for initial differences.

Both samples increased interactions with family from baseline to follow-up, either by phone or visiting in person. Twenty-nine percent of the CCRC residents at baseline and 38 percent at follow-up spent considerable time interacting with family; for the Massachusetts group the corresponding figures were 62 percent at baseline and 72 percent at follow-up. These increases are not surprising given the deterioration in physical functioning and health which both groups experienced. But there was a sharp contrast in the amount of time which these two populations spent in this activity. The Massachusetts residents were likely to spend considerably more time than CCRC residents chatting on the phone and visiting with their family. Based on the controlled logistic regression analysis, the outcome in favor of the Massachusetts group persisted at follow-up.

At both baseline and at follow-up a significantly larger percentage of the Massachusetts group (95 percent at baseline and 96 percent at follow-up) than of the CCRC residents (86 percent at baseline and 85 percent at follow-up) said they had a confidante. There was no significant change in this response from baseline to follow-up for either sample. When we controlled the differences in baseline characteristics, the Massachusetts group continued to be more likely than CCRC residents to have a confidante at follow-up.

For one of the two informal support measures — the number of informal sources currently providing or available to provide help if needed — there was no significant difference between the samples at baseline (2.43 helpers for the Massachusetts group and 2.49 for the CCRC residents). At follow-up, however, there was a significant difference in favor of the Massachusetts sample: an average of 2.89 helpers compared with 2.13 for the CCRC sample. There was a change from baseline to follow-up for both groups, but the changes in the CCRC and Massachusetts samples were not in the same direction. At follow-up, the Massachusetts residents named a significantly larger number of informal helpers, but CCRC residents named significantly fewer helpers at follow-up than at baseline. Once again, the logistic regression procedure estimated that the difference in outcome at follow-up would remain even after we controlled for initial differences.

With respect to the number of those named at baseline who could be relied on indefinitely if help were needed, the average number named by the CCRC residents (1.05) was significantly lower than the average for the Massachusetts group (1.26). At follow-up, members of both samples named significantly fewer helpers who could be counted on indefinitely than at baseline, with no significant difference between the samples (0.88 helpers for the CCRC sample and 0.86 for the Massachusetts sample). However, the logistic regression estimate indicated that when we controlled baseline differences, the CCRC residents at follow-up would have had more informal helpers who could be relied upon indefinitely than would the Massachusetts residents.

Notwithstanding the decrease at follow-up in the number of helpers who could be counted on indefinitely, a majority of the CCRC residents and a sizable proportion of the Massachusetts group (although not a majority) indicated that they had at least one informal helper who could be relied upon to take care of them indefinitely. However, as many as 48 percent of the CCRC sample and 55 percent of the Massachusetts sample felt they had no such person.

The decrease between baseline and follow-up in the number of informal helpers who could be counted on indefinitely for the CCRC sample was in line with the decrease in number of actual helpers; the finding for the Massachusetts elders was not. For them, the number of helpers whom they believed could be relied upon indefinitely had dropped even though the actual number of helpers had increased. It may be that in the absence of a long-term helping relationship with those newly named at follow-up, the elderly person is unsure of the degree to which the helper will be available in the future or if more intensive supports should be needed. The degree and intensity of perceived burden on the informal helpers may also enter the picture.

Although both the Massachusetts and CCRC sample members may have perceived increased dependence upon the informal support system as burdensome, the types and intensity of informal services were likely to differ. Insecurity about continued help from family and friends may grow as service needs become more intense. Compared with the CCRC residents, the types of service and the actual experience of the Massachusetts elders in receiving needed help, usually from family members, may lead them to question how long their loved ones will be able or willing to continue providing such help, particularly as their need for services increases.

Inner Resource and Unmet Needs

This domain consisted of three variables: whether the residents made decisions alone or depended on others; whether they felt they had enough money to live on; and the number of needs that the residents said were unmet. Table 4.5 describes the results of the t-test, the paired t-test, and logistic regression procedures.

Although the vast majority in both samples reported that they made their own decisions at each period of time, both samples were slightly more dependent in decision making at follow-up (more than 95 percent at baseline and more than 90 percent at follow-up). At both points in time, a significantly larger percent of the CCRC sample than the Massachusetts sample made this claim. However, the controlled analyses eliminated the difference found at follow-up; the difference can be explained by baseline differences in the characteristics of the individuals in the two samples rather than environmental factors.

Little change occurred in the proportions saying they had enough money to live on without any trouble. All the same, at both points in time significantly more CCRC residents (88 percent at baseline and 87 percent at follow-up) than Massachusetts residents (63 percent at baseline and 64 percent at follow-up) were in this position. Even after we controlled for initial differences in these two samples, the outcome at follow-up remained the same.

Both CCRC and Massachusetts traditional-community residents reported few unmet needs at baseline and at follow-up, with the average number of self-reported unmet needs considerably less than one. Although the levels of unmet needs rose in both samples, large proportions in both populations said they had none (91 percent of the CCRC sample and 95 percent of the Massachusetts sample at baseline and 86 and 91 percent, respectively, at follow-up). At each point in time, the Massachusetts sample reported significantly fewer unmet needs than did the CCRC residents (0.069 compared with 0.136 for the CCRC sample at baseline and 0.129 compared with 0.218 for the CCRC sample at follow-up).

The controlled analyses, however, reversed this finding. According to the logistic regression estimate, when we controlled baseline characteristics, the CCRC rather than the Massachusetts residents were likely to have had fewer unmet needs. Interestingly, the logistic procedures revealed that the major adjusting variables included living alone/not alone, number of children nearby, and number of limiting medical problems, all of which are conceptually related to unmet needs.

Table 4.5 Inner resource and unmet needs

Variable	Comparison of CCRC vs. MA elderly		Change from baseline to follow-up		Follow-up scores estimated by logistic regression[a]
	Baseline	Follow-up	CCRC sample	MA sample	
Make own decision	CCRC residents were more independent	CCRC residents were more independent	Were less independent	Were less independent	No difference
Enough money to live on	CCRC residents had fewer unmet needs	CCRC residents had fewer unmet needs	No change	No change	CCRC residents would have had fewer unmet needs
No. of unmet needs	MA elderly had fewer unmet needs	MA elderly had fewer unmet needs	More unmet needs	More unmet needs	CCRC residents would have had fewer unmet needs

[a]Logistic regression for ordinal categories.

Conclusions and Insights

At the beginning of this chapter, we raised issues concerning the quality-of-life outcomes:

- the extent to which CCRC residents were similar or different from their age peers in the general community at baseline and at follow-up;
- the nature of changes in the two populations;
- how the CCRC residents would likely have fared at follow-up compared with traditional-community residents when we considered key selection biases predictive of group membership, their baseline scores, and time between baseline and follow-up.

Clearly, as exemplified by the ability to predict the sample membership 86 percent of the time based on a discriminant function equation using just nine variables, CCRC residents were very different from their age peers in the traditional community. They were older, more likely to be female, had achieved higher levels of education, were better off economically, were more likely to live alone, had fewer children nearby, were less likely to have a spouse among their informal helpers, and had a greater number of limiting medical problems; however, they were more able to do their own shopping and perform small errands.

Keeping this in mind, we were not surprised to find many differences between the two populations in outcome variables at both baseline and follow-up. We found significant consistent baseline and follow-up differences for fourteen (88 percent) of the seventeen variables. To a large extent, then, these differences persisted, although sometimes they disappeared when we controlled key baseline characteristics.

As summarized below, for eleven of these fourteen variables, the nature of the change (or lack of change) was also the same. Baseline to follow-up findings were also consistent for an additional three variables. We observed no differences between the samples either at baseline or follow-up for one of these, mental status, and no differential outcome at follow-up was indicated even after controlling for key baseline differences between the two samples.

The nature of the change over time was similar for all eight of the health and functional status (mental and physical) variables; both samples deteriorated somewhat between these periods of time. However, this does not mean that either population had become seriously impaired. Despite deterioration, the majority at follow-up in both samples, often more than 80 percent, gave the most positive or highest quality-of-life response to most of the variables for which deterioration had occurred. Among the individual items of the functional status scales, the only exception was the ability to perform such chores as hanging curtains and washing floors and walls, with fewer than one quarter of the CCRC sample and fewer than one third of the Massachusetts sample saying they could perform such tasks without help.

Although very large percentages of both populations were functionally intact at both baseline and follow-up, at both points in time the CCRC residents perceived their health to be better than did the Massachusetts sample. On average they had higher self-reported ratings of general health, reported less pain, and were less likely to say that sickness or pain had kept them from desired activities. In fact, on average they were more self-sufficient, had fewer ADL and IADL impairments, and were more mobile than the elderly Massachusetts residents. However, except for IADL impairments, all of the follow-up differences between the two samples were eliminated in the analyses that controlled for key baseline differences and time between baseline and follow-up.

We also observed consistent differences between the samples at baseline and at follow-up for seven of the nine remaining variables. Four of these were in favor of the CCRC residents. They were more likely to go out of the house more than once a week; they spent considerably more time than traditional-community residents phoning or visiting friends; they were more independent in decision making; and they were more likely to have enough money to live on without trouble. Except for independence in decision making, the logistic regression procedures estimated that all of these differences in outcome at follow-up would remain, even after controlling for key baseline differences between these two samples.

The remaining three consistent differences were in favor of the Massachusetts sample. They spent more time visiting or phoning family members, more of them said they had a confidante, and they had fewer unmet needs. Although no change was observed from baseline to follow-up in the percentage who had a confidante, the CCRC as well as the Massachusetts residents spent more time interacting with family. The number of unmet needs increased in both samples. All the same, for two of these variables — interacting with family and having a confidante — the follow-up differences between the two samples remained even after controlling for key differences at baseline. However, when we controlled baseline characteristics, it appeared that the CCRC residents would be likely to have had fewer unmet needs than the Massachusetts sample.

Baseline and follow-up findings were not consistent for two somewhat related variables: the number of current informal helpers and the number who could be relied upon indefinitely. The Massachusetts sample had more informal helpers at follow-up than at baseline, whereas the CCRC residents had fewer; the logistic regression procedures indicated that this follow-up difference would remain even when we controlled key differences in baseline characteristics. At follow-up, both samples named fewer persons who could be counted on to provide help indefinitely than they had at baseline, and the differences between the samples were not significant. In this case, however, the logistic regression procedures estimated that, if we adjusted for differences in key baseline characteristics, the CCRC residents would have had more helpers.

The increase in the number of informal helpers which occurred for the Massachusetts sample coincided with deterioration in health and functional status and an expansion in time spent phoning and visiting with family. Presumably the increase in the number of informal helpers was a response to increased need. On the other hand, although the frequency of phoning and visiting family had increased by follow-up for CCRC residents, as a group they had experienced a reduction in the number of informal helpers. Part of this reduction may be attributable to the type of informal helper upon whom CCRC residents often depend.

In fact, exploration of the types of people who helped indicated that almost twice as many of the CCRC residents (45 percent) compared with the Massachusetts residents (23 percent) counted friends and neighbors among their informal helpers. Although the data did not differentiate between types, quantity, and intensity of help that neighbors and friends vs. family members provided, we hypothesized that the repertoire of helping behavior is more limited for friends and neighbors compared with family, perhaps focusing on help with shopping, performing small errands, and transportation services.

To the extent that needs changed, requiring more help with basic ADLs—for example, in dressing, bathing, and toileting—the residents might no longer call upon friends and neighbors to help. Recall also that the CCRC sample members were less likely than the Massachusetts sample to have children living within a one-hour drive—children who would have been more likely than friends and neighbors to step in and help. Instead, since access to needed ancillary services was a major motivating force for entrance to a CCRC, residents may have been counting on and receiving supportive services from this source in response to increased need rather than from informal helpers.

The findings from the controlled analyses are provocative, suggesting insights as to the ways in which the environment affects outcome. In all, differential outcome at follow-up appears to have occurred for nine of the seventeen variables. Six (two thirds) were in favor of the CCRC residents: ability to perform IADL tasks, frequency of going out of the house, frequency of interactions with friends, the number of informal helpers who could be relied upon indefinitely, the extent to which the sample member had enough money to live on without any trouble, and the number of unmet needs. The three variables in which differential outcome occurred in favor of the Massachusetts residents were: interactions with family, having a confidante, and the number of informal helpers (although not the number they believed could be relied upon indefinitely).

These findings suggest that the variables in which differential outcome (after adjustment) favors the Massachusetts group are connected in one way or another to family ties and to some extent may be a function of differential expectations of these two populations and the opportunities afforded by their respective environments. The differences both in time spent phoning or visiting with family and in having a confidante, which favor the traditional-community residents, may in fact be a natural effect of living in these different environments. Increasing frailty among elderly traditional-community residents may engender greater expectation regarding interactions with and services from family members than would be demanded by CCRC residents or expected in the CCRC environment. Many elderly traditional-community residents either live close to or move in with family members based on their need for supportive services, facilitating increased contact and the development of intimate relationships. Furthermore, having someone close and the importance of that relationship may be major variables determining whether a person chooses a living arrangement such as a CCRC. The different responses by the samples to both of these variables may also reflect group personality and philosophical disparities.

Similarly, features of the CCRC environment may in fact have been instrumental in bringing about each of the results favoring the residents of these communities. The differential outcome in interactions with friends in favor of the CCRC resident is in an expected direction, given the nature of the CCRC environment. The proximity of more people of similar age and interests can be considered an advantage of CCRC living over residence in the traditional community. Furthermore, the increase from baseline to follow-up in time spent in this activity indicates that CCRC members may have expanded their network of friends. Because of the opportunities for social interaction within the CCRC itself, deteriorating health does not seem to deter CCRC residents from increased interaction with friends or, for that matter, from going out of the house, but it does appear to do so for persons living in the traditional community.

In addition, the differential outcome regarding ability to perform

IADL tasks appears at least in part to be a function of the environmental demands of the two populations. As we discussed previously, CCRCs provide many services such as light housekeeping, meal preparation, and transportation. Particularly pertinent to shopping, doing small errands, and similar tasks, CCRC residents require less energy to negotiate the environment than that required by their age peers in the traditional community. The CCRC residents might thus have more residual energy to perform IADL tasks when necessary, and their health and problems in physical functioning may be less likely to affect their ability to participate in other activities as well as to perform necessary tasks. The CCRC services might also give residents more free time to participate in leisure activities and to go out of the house more often than persons like themselves in the traditional community.

The CCRC services undoubtedly have implications as well for the types and intensity of services that residents expect from informal helpers. Taking into consideration that a major motivation for joining a CCRC was access to needed services, presumably members of the CCRC sample turned to the CCRC rather than to family and friends as their needs became more severe. In any event, help with activities such as meal preparation and housekeeping tended to be part of the services provided by the CCRC; furthermore, some CCRCs offered personal care as part of their on-site amenities.

For impaired elderly persons in traditional-community settings, informal helpers (usually spouses and children) are likely to provide such services. Both the Massachusetts and CCRC sample members may perceive increased dependence upon the informal support system as burdensome to their informal helpers. But the types and intensity of informal services and the experience of the Massachusetts sample in receiving them make them more likely than the CCRC residents to perceive that the care provided to them is burdensome (often very burdensome) to their informal helpers. To the extent that insecurity accompanies added reliance on informal sources for needed services, this insecurity might thus be relatively less pronounced in the CCRC sample. When we consider differences in initial functional status and informal support variables, particularly the baseline measure of these variables, this insecurity translates into a relatively greater reduction in the perception by the Massachusetts compared with the CCRC sample members of how many helpers could be counted on indefinitely, or as long as needed, should they become sick.

The logistic regression finding regarding the number of unmet needs is interesting. It indicates that major baseline differences accounted for the differences at follow-up in unmet needs in favor of the Massachusetts sample; that is, if the two samples had been more alike on these characteristics (e.g., having more children nearby), the CCRC residents would actually have done better. Nevertheless, traditional-community residents appear to be more likely to have relationships with children and other loved ones which tend to engender sensitivity and enhance response to increased need. The issues of sensitivity to changing needs of residents and the enhancement of timely response are important areas of concern for CCRC operators.

Finally, CCRC residents were likely to say they had enough money to live on without any trouble and to interact more frequently with friends than did the Massachusetts sample. The finding that even after adjustment for baseline differences, the CCRC residents were more likely to say they had enough money to live on supports the CCRC advocate argument that the CCRC environment affords greater security than that of the traditional community. It may be that given the assurance of access and in many cases security as to the ability to cover long-term care services with little additional cost, equal amounts of money to live on are more likely to be considered "enough" in a CCRC than elsewhere.

FIVE

Use of Medicare-Covered Medical Care by CCRC Residents

CCRCs can potentially affect the way their residents use the services available to them. Implicit within the CCRC concept is immediate access to a range of services. Staff can refer residents to facility- or community-based programs and services that specifically address their needs. Some CCRCs have on-site medical offices or clinics that might encourage or facilitate residents' use of medical services. Furthermore, CCRCs have nursing home units close by and might also have personal care units and/or services that provide a continuum of care between independent living and institutional residence. The availability of these services could impact on residents' use of costly hospital inpatient care.

Despite the interest that social planners and federal and state policy makers have in the CCRC concept, there are very few hard data on this housing and service delivery arrangement. With the exception of studies of nursing homes (Cohen 1988; Cohen et al. 1988b), no study has assessed how CCRC residents use medical care in a typical year or in their last year of life compared with such use by elderly residents of more traditional-community settings. One might predict that because CCRC services are available, residents might replace Medicare-covered services with the social services and noncovered long-term care services that the CCRC supplies. Alternately, CCRCs might be able to substitute Medicare-reimbursable skilled medical services for less intensive non — Medicare-covered services, thereby increasing the utilization of medical care services covered by the Medicare program. In this chapter we present research to clarify the effect of CCRC living on the use of Medicare-covered medical services.

Data and Methods
Selecting the Study Sample

As we pointed out in Chapter 1, we drew a sample of nineteen CCRCs from the four geographic areas with the largest concentration of these facilities: Arizona, Florida, Pennsylvania, and southern California.

Much of this chapter was reported in Ruchlin et al. (1993).

Nine of these study sites offered extended contracts, and ten offered limited contracts. In addition to providing access to a nursing home, ten sites had personal care units that furnished special assistance with activities of daily living (ADLs).

The first of two analyses in this chapter focuses on the representative random samples of CCRC residents and traditional-community residents (as described in Chapter 1) who completed baseline interviews and for whom follow-up information was available. In some cases, we interviewed a resident proxy if the resident had become too disabled to participate in an interview or had died between baseline and follow-up. We gathered data on medical service utilization and costs for each person for a one-year period beginning with his or her entry into the study.

CCRC residents eligible for inclusion in the second analysis, which focused on the resident's last year of life, included the first thirty-three people in each facility who had died in 1985 plus everyone in the representative random sample who had died between the baseline and follow-up interviews. The study period for the death sample consisted of the twelve months before death.

To assess patterns of resource use, we compared a sample of individuals first interviewed in 1982 as part of a longitudinal study of a representative sample of elderly traditional-community Massachusetts residents. That study had been conducted by the Social Gerontological Research Division of the Research and Training Institute of the Hebrew Rehabilitation Center for Aged (HRCA).[1] To match the period covered by the CCRC study, we selected data for the comparison sample from a twelve-month period, from 1986 to 1987.

The main study sample consisted of 1,666 CCRC residents and 1,379 elderly traditional-community residents. For the last-year-of-life

1. The cost of gathering a special comparison sample for this study would have been prohibitive. We could have used either an existing national or regional (i.e., Massachusetts) data set. Neither would have been directly comparable to the four states represented in the CCRC sample. We selected the available regional data set as its contents, methods of data collection, and recall period (twelve months) more closely resembled the data collected for the study's CCRC sample. The Massachusetts and CCRC data-gathering instruments encompassed the same utilization elements, data-gathering staff were subject to the same training protocols, and the same protocol was used to obtain data from proxies when the respondent could not provide information because of a physical or cognitive problem. Data for the CCRC sample were gathered through personal interviews; telephone interviews were used for gathering data for the Massachusetts sample. For both samples, telephone interviews were used to gather data from proxies for decedents. A small proportion of each sample (9 percent of the original CCRC sample and 4 percent of the original Massachusetts sample) refused to complete the follow-up survey. An additional 4.6 percent of the CCRC sample could not be located at follow-up.

sample, we obtained the necessary follow-up data for 364 CCRC residents and 464 traditional-community residents.[2] To assess service utilization differences over a uniform-sized sample and to preserve all of the available degrees of freedom for the statistical analyses, we weighted the CCRC and traditional-community samples to the size of 1,552 and 414, respectively.

Service Use and Cost Data

In the ensuing analyses we focused exclusively on services and costs that the Medicare program incurred. We did not include the utilization and costs of formal and informal community-based personal care services or other services not covered by Medicare.

We obtained Medicare identification numbers from the sample members and utilization and expenditure data from the Health Care Financing Administration (HCFA) Medicare Automated Data Retrieval System (MADRS) Part A-Part B skeleton file. In generating the hospital payment variable, we factored in adjustments to the initial payment as well as payments for direct and indirect medical education costs, capital costs, bad debts, and having a disproportionate share of indigent patients. Specific utilization data (admissions and length of stay and visits) were available only for services covered by Medicare Part A. Payment data only were available for services covered by Medicare Part B, specifically ambulatory medical care.

We gathered detailed self-report data on socioeconomic and functional status and medical care utilization in the sample surveys by HRCA researchers. We validated the self-reported information on hospital and nursing home admission and length of stay by contacting these facilities directly. We used this information to proxy for missing data and to adjust the utilization and expenditure profiles for external factors. For individuals in the death sample, proxy[3] respondents replaced the self-reported data.

Proxying for Missing Data

For the main analysis, Medicare identification numbers were unavailable for 41 CCRC residents (2.5 percent of the overall sample) and

2. The overall death rates for both samples were comparable: 6.4 percent for the CCRC sample and 7.3 percent for the Massachusetts sample.

3. Sixty-eight percent of the proxy respondents for the CCRC group and 74 percent of the proxy respondents for the traditional-community residence group were either spouses, daughters, sons, daughters-in-law, or sons-in-law. Five percent of the proxy respondents in each sample were either friends, neighbors, or formal care providers. The balance were other relatives.

339 traditional-community residents (24.6 percent of this sample). We employed statistical techniques to predict which of these individuals would use medical care and how much they would use. We made two adjustments to the MADRS physician use data to correct for suspected data misclassification and underreporting. See Ruchlin et al. (1993) for details of the proxying process and data adjustments.

We were able to obtain Medicare identification numbers for only eighty-seven CCRC residents in the last-year-of-life sample (24 percent of the CCRC death sample). Consequently, we used self-reported medical care use data and constant-dollar shadow prices for both the CCRC and non — CCRC resident samples for this part of the analysis. We relied on average hospital payments per admission, derived from the available MADRS data for the CCRC and non — CCRC samples, and state-specific 1986 Medicaid per diem nursing home rates to convert self-reported use data into expenditure data. Utilization rates reflecting the utilization of home health care and physician care were not available from the self-reported data. Thus, we did not include this information in the death analysis. Furthermore, in the death sample we did not attempt to exclude nursing home use not covered by Medicare.

Adjusting for External Factors

We adjusted utilization and expenditure profiles to control for the effects of personal characteristics and geographic resource availability and cost differences unique to each of the study samples. Based on discriminant function analysis, the following were the personal characteristic variables that differentiated between the two groups for whom baseline data had been gathered (the main analysis): age, sex, number of children living nearby, income level, years of schooling, number of limiting medical problems, ability to do shopping and errands, whether a spouse provided help or could be relied on to provide help, and living alone/not alone. For the last-year-of-life analysis, the variables identified were age, sex, orientation to time and place (twelve months before death), and ability to do personal care.

To control further for individual health status and tendency to use medical care, we also used a variable indicating self-reported use of that service in the year before the initial interview. Medical care utilization levels are fairly consistent over time (see, e.g., Anderson and Knickman 1984; Densen et al. 1959; McCall and Wai 1983; Mossey and Shapiro 1985), suggesting that the premeasures are good health status proxies. Because a direct premeasure for inpatient physician care and home health care was not available, inpatient hospital use became the proxy for inpatient physician care, and the amount of (self-reported) personal care became the proxy for home health care. For the last-year-of-life analysis, we added a variable that indicated whether the person was in a community or institutional setting twelve months before death.

We abstracted selected county-level data from the 1986 Area Resource File (ARF) compiled by the U.S. Department of Health and Human Services, Bureau of Health Professions. ARF data controlled for resource availability and, in the case of physician care, for area-specific charge levels as well. The ARF variables we selected were per capita income (all services), number of physicians/thousand population (hospital care, home health care, and physician visits), inpatient beds/thousand population (hospital and nursing home care), hospital occupancy rate for medical/surgical beds (hospital, nursing home, and home health care), and the prevailing charge index for generalists and specialists combined (physician care). We had considered total nursing home beds/thousand population above the age of 65 but eventually dropped it because it totally defined the sample.

We used a multivariate analysis of variance and covariance (MANOVA) to generate the adjusted variable values reported below.[4] Given the small number of people ($N = 26$) utilizing Medicare-covered nursing home care, and as a result the limited degrees of freedom, we could not use as covariates all of the potential personal characteristics, ARF, and health premeasure variables in the main analysis. We therefore used a two-step process to select the two most important covariates for the MANOVA program. First, for each aspect of nursing home care we generated a zero-order correlation matrix and selected the variable with the highest correlation. Second, we produced a partial correlation matrix controlling for the variable that was just designated and selected the variable with the highest correlation in this set, yielding two covariates for the MANOVAs.

The resulting covariates were as follows:

- for any nursing home admission: age and number of limiting health conditions;
- for number of nursing home admissions: total inpatient beds/thousand population and family income;
- for total payment for nursing home care: per capita income and ability to do small errands;

---

4. Logistic regressions were also run to derive predicted values for the any-use variables and thus check the accuracy of the MANOVA values, which do not embody a logistic regression specification. The adjusted values generated by this process were quite comparable to those generated by the MANOVAs and are not reported here.

▪ for payment per nursing home admission: number of limiting conditions and living alone/not alone.

Data Presentation

We report here service utilization and expenditure data for both "utilizers" and the entire study samples. The utilizer data reflect only the experience of sample members who used that type of care. The sample profiles also included those individuals with no service utilization in the denominators. Although the utilizer profiles are interesting from a perspective of medical care use, the results in the sample columns form the basis for assessing overall economic difference. Expenditure data in the main analysis spanned a multiyear period. We converted all expenditures to base-year (1985–86) levels by employing a 6 percent discount rate. In addition, we assessed the sensitivity of the findings to the selection of a particular discount rate using three alternate rates: 4, 8, and 10 percent. Constant-dollar shadow prices in the last-year-of-life analysis obviated the need for discounting in this aspect of the study.

Findings

Characteristics of the Study Samples

From a sociodemographic perspective, there were significant differences between CCRC residents and non – CCRC residents in the main analysis. As shown in Table 5.1, the CCRC residents were older, had a higher representation of females, and had higher income levels and educational attainment.

In this sample (which included people who died) not only did more of the CCRC residents have limiting health problems (44.1 vs. 39.6 percent), but more also had instrumental activities of daily living (IADL) limitations than did the elderly traditional-community residents: 8.9 percent of CCRC residents compared with 11.5 percent of the Massachusetts sample had one or more IADL limitations. Only limited sociodemographic data were available for members of the death sample, but they indicated that there were also differences between both of the study samples.

Service Utilization and Expenditure Profiles (Main Analysis)

Hospital Care. The average cost per admission for both groups was in the $4,400-$4,900 range. Approximately 18 percent of both samples reported that they had some hospital care during the twelve-month study period (see Table 5.2). Of those who had a hospital admission (i.e.,

Table 5.1 Characteristics of the study samples

Sample characteristic	Main analysis sample		Death sample	
	CCRC	Community	CCRC	Community
Age in years	81.8	77.8[a]	84.5	84.5
	(5.6)	(5.9)	(6.3)	(6.3)
Female (%)	75.0	60.7[a]	68.4	60.9[b]
	(43.3)	(48.9)	(46.5)	(48.9)
Married (%)	40.2	41.4		
	(49.0)	(49.3)		
Income (% <$20,000)	22.3	66.9[a]		
	(41.7)	(47.1)		
Education (% high school graduate)	89.7	46.1[a]	84.2	43.3[a]
	(30.4)	(50.0)	(36.5)	(49.6)
Medical problems (% with one or more limiting conditions)	44.1	39.6[a]		
	(49.7)	(48.9)		
ADL limitations (% with one or more)	8.9	11.5[b]		
	(28.5)	(31.9)		
IADL limitations (% with one or more)	58.1	47.8[a]		
	(49.3)	(50.0)		
N	1,552	1,552	414	414

Note. Standard deviations are in parentheses.
[a]Statistically significant at $p \leq 0.01$.
[b]Statistically significant at $p \leq 0.05$.

utilizers), elderly traditional-community residents had a greater number of admissions per year than did CCRC residents (1.70 vs. 1.43). Traditional-community residents who had been hospitalized also reported more days in the hospital during the study year than did the CCRC residents (sixteen vs. twelve days), but this difference lacked statistical significance at conventional levels. Because of the greater number of admissions per year, average Medicare payments (cost) per utilizer were higher in the traditional-community resident sample than in the CCRC sample ($8,200 vs. $6,882), although this difference failed to attain statistical significance.

When viewed from the perspective of the entire sample, fairly comparable hospital admissions per year (0.32 vs. 0.26) and covered-day (3 vs. 2.3) profiles appeared. Although a 20 percent differential emerged with regard to average annual Medicare expenditures ($1,533 vs. $1,277), this difference was not statistically significant even at a relaxed threshold of $p = 0.10$.

Table 5.2 CCRC vs. community residence samples: Medicare-covered hospital utilization profiles

Variable	Utilizers		Sample	
	CCRC	Community	CCRC	Community
Any hospital care (%)	18.28	18.78		
Average no. of admissions	1.43	1.70[a]	0.26	0.32
Average no. of covered days	12.20	16.06	2.33	2.98
Average Medicare payment	$6,882	$8,200	$1,277	$1,533
Average payment per admission	$4,873	$4,418		

[a]Differences were statistically significant at $p \leq 0.05$.

Nursing Home Care[5]. Very few people in either sample used Medicare-approved nursing home care during the twelve-month study period. As shown in Table 5.3, only 1.3 percent of the CCRC sample and 0.4 percent of the community-based sample reported any use of Medicare-covered nursing home care. For those who did use this type of care in each sample (i.e., the utilizers), no statistically significant differences emerged at $p = 0.05$ or lower. The average number of admissions was slightly greater than one, and the average number of Medicare-covered nursing home days ranged from nineteen to fifty. Average expenditure per admission was less in the CCRC sample ($1,309 vs. $3,139) but over the entire twelve-month exposure period, average total expenditures were not significantly different ($1,844 vs. $2,901).

When viewed from the perspective of the entire sample, a large difference in nursing home utilization appeared, even though a comparable difference in hospital use was not found. In addition to having more people with a Medicare-covered nursing home stay than the traditional-community sample had, the CCRC sample also had on average more admissions during the year (0.02 vs. 0.001) and more Medicare-covered days (0.47 vs. 0.01). Medicare payments per sample member were also higher for the CCRC group ($27 vs. $3).

Home Health Care. Eighty-eight elderly traditional-community residents and twenty-three CCRC residents received Medicare-covered

5. The nursing homes in five of the nineteen CCRCs were not Medicare certified. None of the 374 residents of these facilities included in this study had any Medicare-covered nursing home admissions. A review of their self-reported data uncovered two nursing home admissions among this group. The nature of these admissions is not known. Their exclusion from the analysis reported here does not affect the overall direction of the findings reported in this section.

Table 5.3 CCRC vs. community residence samples: Medicare-covered nursing home utilization profiles

Variable	Utilizers		Sample	
	CCRC	Community	CCRC	Community
Any nursing home care (%)			1.31	0.37[a]
Average no. of admissions	1.20	1.12	0.02	0.001[a]
Average no. of covered days	39.68	18.53	0.47	0.01[a]
Average Medicare payment	$1,844	$2,901	$27	$3[a]
Average payment per admission	$1,309	$3,139		

[a]Differences were statistically significant at $p \leq 0.01$.

Table 5.4 CCRC vs. community residence samples: Medicare-covered home health care utilization profiles

Variable	Utilizers		Sample	
	CCRC	Community	CCRC	Community
Any home health care (%)			1.69	5.51[a]
Average no. of visits	19.23	21.76	0.33	0.93
Average Medicare payment	$774	$833	$13	$35
Average payment per visit	$45	$37[b]		

[a]Differences were statistically significant at $p \leq 0.01$.
[b]Differences were statistically significant at $p \leq 0.05$.

home health care. There was no statistically significant difference (see Table 5.4) among those who did use this service in the annual number of visits (approximately twenty) or average Medicare payments (approximately $800). The average payment per visit, however, was higher in the CCRC sample ($45 vs. $37).

On a samplewide basis, only one significant difference emerged: the overall use rate noted above. Despite the relatively high differential in the average number of visits (0.33 vs. 0.93) and the average payments ($13 vs. $35), these differentials lacked statistical significance at conventional levels.

Physician Care. Average annual payments for inpatient physician care among those who had a hospital stay ranged from $1,200 to $1,290 for both groups. When we allocated these costs over the entire sample, the average expenditure for physician inpatient care ranged from $220 to $237 (see Table 5.5).

Table 5.5 CCRC vs. community residence samples: Medicare-covered physician care utilization profiles

Variable	Utilizers		Sample	
	CCRC	Community	CCRC	Community
In hospital				
% with bills			17.94	19.13
Average payment	$1,202	$1,288	$221	$237
In nursing home				
% with bills			19.71	1.87[a]
Average payment	$117	$275[a]	$46	$5[a]
Ambulatory medical care				
% with bills			97.10	84.67[a]
Average payment	$297	$501[a]	$284	$430[a]

[a]Differences were statistically significant at $p \leq 0.01$.

We found a significant difference for physician care rendered in a nursing home setting. Twenty percent of the CCRC resident sample had bills for this service compared with only 2 percent of the traditional-community residents. Average Medicare payments were much higher for the latter group using physician services than for those in the CCRC ($275 vs. $117). However, when we averaged these payments over the entire sample, a $46 vs. $5 profile emerged in favor of the traditional-community residence group.

Ninety-seven percent of the CCRC sample and 85 percent of the traditional-community residence sample incurred physician bills for ambulatory medical care. For those with such bills, the average annual payments were $297 for the CCRC residents and $501 for the traditional-community residents. At the samplewide level, annual expenditures were $284 and $430, respectively, for the CCRC and community samples.

All Medicare-Covered Services. Ninety-six percent of CCRC residents and 86 percent of the traditional-community residents used at least one Medicare-covered service during the twelve-month study (see Table 5.6). Among the utilizers, average annual Medicare expenditures were $1,936 for CCRC residents compared with $2,625 for non—CCRC residents. When we spread this utilization over the entire sample, the resulting averages were $1,772 and $2,312, a differential that attains statistical significance only at a relaxed threshold of $p = 0.09$. Within the

Table 5.6 CCRC vs. community residence samples: Total Medicare
expenditures

Variable	Utilizers		Sample	
	CCRC	Community	CCRC	Community
Any utilization (%)			95.92	86.18[a]
Average expenditure (6% discounting)	$1,936	$2,625[b]	$1,772	$2,312
Average expenditure (4% discounting)	$1,958	$2,686[b]	$1,791	$2,365
Average expenditure (8% discounting)	$1,914	$2,567[b]	$1,753	$2,262
Average expenditure (10% discounting)	$1,893	$2,512	$1,736	$2,214

[a]Differences were statistically significant at $p \leq 0.01$.
[b]Differences were statistically significant at $p \leq 0.05$.

CCRC sector, no significant differences emerged when the data were disaggregated into the four geographic regions from which the CCRC sample was drawn.

Using a 4, 8, or 10 percent discount rate affected the findings only minimally. Only at a 10 percent discount rate did the difference for the utilizer groups fail to attain significance at the conventional threshold of $p = 0.05$. At the sample level, using a 4 or 8 percent discount rate led to a significant finding only at a relaxed threshold of $p = 0.08$ or 0.10, respectively.

Use of Institutional Care in the Last Year of Life

Hospital Care. As reported in Table 5.7, a greater proportion of the traditional-community residence sample than of the CCRC sample used hospital care in their last year of life (78 vs. 52 percent). Although non–CCRC residents using hospital care appeared to have had, on average, more admissions during this period (1.81 vs. 1.47), longer stays (thirty-five vs. twenty days), and higher estimated expenditures for care ($8,997 vs. $7,910), none of these differences was statistically significant at conventional levels. However, when we viewed this utilization from a samplewide perspective, statistically significant differences favoring the CCRC sample emerged. As a group, these individuals had fewer admissions in the study year (0.75 vs. 1.41), fewer days of care (10 vs. 26), and lower estimated average expenditures ($3,854 vs. $7,268).

Table 5.7 CCRC vs. community residence samples: Self-reported utilization and expenditures for institutional care in the year before death

Variable	Utilizers		Death sample	
	CCRC	Community	CCRC	Community
Hospital care				
% with use			51.84	77.85[a]
Average no. of admissions	1.47	1.81	0.75	1.41[a]
Average no. of days	19.52	34.61	9.76	26.31[a]
Average payment	$7,910	$8,997	$3,854	$7,268[a]
Nursing home care				
% with use			65.89	36.42[a]
Average no. of days	181.07	189.68	118.01	69.40[a]
Average payment	$8,526	$9,669	$5,565	$3,533[a]
Total institutional care				
% with use			83.72	85.47
Average no. of days	150.96	113.33[b]		
	127.83	95.69[a]		
Average payment	$11,495	$12,490[a]	$9,485	$10,746[a]

[a]Differences were statistically significant at $p \leq 0.01$.

[b]Differences were statistically significant at $p \leq 0.05$.

Nursing Home Care. We noted a different pattern for the use of nursing home care. More people in CCRCs than in the traditional community were in a skilled or intermediate care facility during their last year of life (66 vs. 36 percent). Although we found no statistically significant differences with regard to either the amount of or the estimated expenditures for nursing home care utilizers, significant sample level differences did emerge. On average, CCRC residents used 118 days of nursing home care compared with 69 days for traditional-community residents. Expenditures for nursing home care were also higher in the CCRC group ($5,565 vs. $3,533).

All Institutional Care. When we aggregated across both types of institutional care (e.g., hospitals and nursing homes), approximately 85 percent of each sample used some type of institutional care in their last year of life. Although CCRC residents used more total days of care (128 vs. 96) they generated lower samplewide aggregate expenditures ($9,485 vs. $10,746).

Summary and Discussion

The data in this chapter indicated that for an average year at the samplewide level, living in a CCRC was not associated with significantly lower annual expenditures for Medicare-covered medical care services. Although the CCRC resident sample incurred about $540 less in annual expenditures than the traditional-community residents ($1,772 vs. $2,312), this difference was not statistically significant at even a relaxed threshold of $p = 0.10$. Submerged within this overall finding were two others worthy of note. A larger percent of CCRC than traditional-community residents reported some use of medical care services during the twelve-month period (96 vs. 86 percent), but, for those with any utilization, individuals living in a CCRC experienced, on average, lower expenditures ($1,936 vs. $2,625). The net effect of these two findings was overall samplewide patterns that were not significantly different.

In both settings, inpatient hospital care accounted for approximately 70 percent of total expenditures. Very few sample members in either setting used Medicare-covered skilled nursing home or home health care. These services, when combined, accounted for less than 2 percent of overall annual expenditures. Statistically significant expenditure differences, at the sample level, appeared for only one of these services: skilled nursing home care. More individuals residing in CCRCs used this service than did people living in traditional-community settings (1.2 vs. 0.3 percent), and they had higher average annual costs ($27 vs. $3). Cohen (1988) and Cohen et al. (1988b) reported similar findings with regard to nursing home care.

CCRC residents incurred higher annual samplewide expenditures for physician care provided in a nursing home setting ($46 vs. $5) but lower expenditures for ambulatory physician care ($284 vs. $430). Expenditures for physician care delivered in a hospital did not differ across settings.

In the aggregate, Medicare-related expenditure and service utilization profiles generally conformed to national patterns. At the specific service level, however, a few notable differences emerged. Over the period covered by this study (1986-87) average Medicare expenditures per enrollee were $2,491 (Helbing et al. 1991).[6] Our estimates as reported in Table 5.6 for the traditional-community residents were somewhat lower,

---

6. Data presented in Helbing et al. (1991) reflect total Medicare program expenditures. Separate data for the aged and disabled population were not reported. Unpublished average Medicare enrollment, provided by HCFA staff for 1986–87, was 32,080,456. This statistic was used to calculate expenditures per enrollee.

but we did not include all Medicare-covered services in this study. CCRC residents had a lower expenditure profile, a pattern consistent with that noted in this study. With regard to the use of inpatient hospital care, the national average number of admissions per enrollee was 0.31. The average payment per admission was $4,262, and the average payment per enrollee was $1,310 (Latta and Keene 1990). Except for the CCRC hospital admission rate, which was lower, the remaining hospital utilization patterns reported in Table 5.2 for both the CCRC and the traditional-community residents were in line with the national data. Similarly, payments for physician care in both study samples resembled the national level of about $600 per year (Helbing et al. 1991).

Nationally, approximately 1 percent of all Medicare enrollees used Medicare-covered skilled nursing home care in 1986–87. Those using this type of care stayed on average 26.1 days and paid on average $2,019 for it. On a per-enrollee basis, 0.26 days were covered, and average payments for care were $20.35 (Silverman 1991). CCRC residents used more days of care but reported lower payments. Members of our traditional-community residence sample used fewer days of care but had higher costs (see Table 5.3). A different pattern emerged with regard to Medicare-covered home health care. Unpublished HCFA data indicated that about 5 percent of all enrollees utilized this care. Those doing so had about twenty-four visits per year and generated total payments of $1,119. Use of home health care services by members of the traditional-community residence sample generally conformed to this national pattern. There was a much lower utilization profile within our CCRC sample (see Table 5.4).

In assessing the service utilization and expenditure findings reported in this study, one must remember that we limited the scope of the analysis to services and expenditures relevant to the Medicare program. The impact of CCRC living on non — Medicare-covered nursing home and home health care and on the use of both formal and informal community-based social services remains to be explored. Similarly, we did not include in this analysis out-of-pocket payments to cover deductibles, copayments, and fees that exceeded Medicare's customary, prevailing, and reasonable threshold. It is possible that when the analysis is broadened to encompass these types of care and out-of-pocket payments, a different overall finding could emerge.

We must draw attention to two attributes of the data sets in this study. First, the comparison sample was drawn from only one state (Massachusetts). Given the known regional variation in the use of medical care, one might question whether this selection exerted an independent impact on the results. The total Medicare expenditure profile for elderly traditional-community residents in the Massachusetts sample was fairly comparable to the national norm. The same applied for the hospital care and home health care expenditure patterns. However, this was not the case for nursing home care. In the light of the very low use of Medicare-covered nursing home care in both study samples, it is doubtful whether our use of the Massachusetts data set as our comparison group introduced any significant bias.

Also noteworthy is that the CCRC and traditional-community samples were not comparable with regard to sociodemographic, health, and functional status. The CCRC sample was better educated, wealthier, and healthier. In the analyses reported in this chapter we sought to control for these (and supply-related) factors. One could question whether we accounted for the full effect of these factors.

The analysis focusing on the last year of life, which was based on self-reported data collected from proxies, indicated that living in a CCRC was associated with lower expenditures for hospital care but higher expenditures for all nursing home care during this period of time. When we combined both hospital and nursing home care into a category of total institutional use, the CCRC sample displayed lower total expenditures. Even with recognition of the origin of the data we used in this aspect of the study, the results do support a hypothesis that residence in a CCRC generates overall medical care cost savings during a person's last year of life. The primary source of these savings would be lower expenditures for hospital care, which accounts for the bulk of Medicare expenditures. Even though CCRC residents used more (Medicare-covered and/or non — Medicare-covered) nursing home care during their last year of life, the savings they reaped from a lesser use of hospital care appeared to be large enough to generate overall savings. Had we been able to exclude non — Medicare-covered nursing home use from this aspect of the study, the estimated savings might have been much larger.

Clearly, we need additional research to test this hypothesis and to extend the scope of the analysis to encompass physician care and home care. Given the fact that hospital costs drive the medical system, there is no reason to predict that broadening the scope of the analysis to include noninstitutional care would dramatically reverse the Medicare-relevant profiles presented here.

SIX

CCRC Residents: A Summary and Conclusions

CCRCs are planned communities for elderly persons which allow residents to age in place. As they have developed in this country, CCRCs are private-sector ventures (most often, but not necessarily, nonprofit) that have depended financially on entrance and monthly fees, incorporating features of pooled risk. As part of a long-term contract with the resident (usually for life), the CCRC provides the resident with housing, amenities, and a range of services, including supportive services and, when necessary, nursing home care. The housing for residents in the independent living units (ILUs, usually apartments, but sometimes town houses or cottages) and the nursing home are generally on the same campus, with residential and nursing care coordinated or managed by the administrator. Although CCRCs vary in the extent to which the entrance and monthly fees for residential care cover nursing home care, the contracts, at a minimum, guarantee access to nursing home care should it be needed; and at a maximum, they cover the full cost of nursing home care.

This guarantee of access to nursing home care along with commitment to the community (long-term contracts involving at least some pooled risk) distinguishes entry-fee CCRCs from rentals. Of the CCRCs studied here, pooled risk existed even in the one facility whose arrangement was almost completely of the fee-for-service type. Residents of this facility who suffer financial reversals or whose economic resources are drained from prolonged care in the facility's health center (nursing home) and are unable to pay the fees (or full fees) for residence or care are not asked to leave. Although such residents were expected to apply for governmental entitlements (e.g., SSI and Medicaid) to help defray the cost of CCRC residence and nursing home care, these mechanisms only partially cover the expenses associated with their care.

This book has focused in particular on residents of these communities. Although demographic information and insights can be gleaned from reports of CCRC operators and from case histories and studies involving one or two facilities, relatively little hard data exist about this population, particularly information gathered from residents of the facilities themselves. The wealth of information and analyses in this book contributes to the literature about this population and is at least a step in filling the gap.

In this book we presented findings from a multifaceted longitudinal study conducted in the mid to late 1980s in which we obtained data directly from almost two thousand residents in nineteen CCRCs in four states (four in Arizona and five each in California, Florida, and Pennsylvania). All of the residents were living in apartments (or other ILUs) when we first contacted them.

Nine of these nineteen communities were extended CCRCs; that is, except for additional charges for meal services not ordinarily included in the monthly fee, these CCRCs provided nursing home care on a virtually unlimited basis at no extra cost to the resident. CCRCs providing less financial protection were considered limited CCRCs, whether they furnished nursing home care on a full fee-for-service basis, a discounted fee-for-service basis, or for a limited period without additional charges before implementing services on a full or discounted fee-for-service basis.

We obtained data about these residents primarily from initial (baseline) interviews with them and follow-up interviews conducted on average sixteen months later. For analyses pertaining to Medicare use, we also gathered data from the Health Care Financing Administration (HCFA) Medicare Automated Data Retrieval System (MADRS) Part A-Part B skeleton file. We looked at both recent (in the CCRC for less than a year) and longer-stay residents of extended and limited CCRCs, comparing their background characteristics, reasons for moving to a CCRC, their activities while a resident, their satisfaction with the CCRC, and attitudes about their own aging and quality-of-life. Comparisons between residents of extended and limited CCRCs included only sample members who were alive at follow-up.

In addition, we gathered similar data from interviews as part of a longitudinal study of a representative sample of elderly Massachusetts traditional-community residents as well as comparable data for the Massachusetts sample derived from HCFA MADRS, and we used data from other secondary sources (e.g., census data) for comparison purposes. We limited comparisons of CCRC residents with the Massachusetts residents to sample members who were at least 70 years old. We compared persons who were alive at follow-up on a series of quality-of-life indicators at baseline and follow-up, on changes between these two points in time, and on outcome at follow-up controlling for key differences in baseline characteristics. We also performed controlled comparisons of the use of medical care (relevant to Medicare), including persons who had died. For a special sample of CCRC and traditional-community residents who had died, we compared their use of and expenditures for medical care during their last year of life. For the last-year-of-life comparison we included in that special sample everyone in the larger samples of CCRC and Massachusetts residents who had died between baseline and follow-up plus the first thirty-three people in each facility who had died in 1985 plus everyone in the longitudinal study of a representative sample of Massachusetts traditional-community residents who had died in 1985.

Key Findings

Supporting the findings by others (AAHA and Ernst and Young 1992; Netting 1991), data from the CCRC study sample members (regardless of age or date of entrance) clearly indicate that the CCRCs tend to serve white, well-educated, middle- to upper-middle-class people from the older segments of the elderly population, the majority of whom are women who are at least 75 years old. The large majority of sample members, including women, had been part of the work force (of the total sample, only 5 percent of the longer-stay and 6 percent of the more recent entrants reported *housewife* as their occupation for most of their lives). More than 85 percent had been white-collar workers, more than half of whom had been professionals.

Age-Stratified Comparisons

Age-stratified comparisons of baseline (when first interviewed) characteristics of CCRC residents age 70 and older with traditional-community residents of this age in the Massachusetts sample indicated key differences between the CCRC and traditional-community residents for each of the age-stratified categories. The two populations age 70 through 74 differed the least.

Demographically, across all age groups, CCRC residents were more likely than the Massachusetts sample to be white, live alone, have fewer children nearby, be better educated, have income from personal investments, and have higher incomes. They were less likely to be Medicaid recipients (almost none were on Medicaid) or to be below the poverty level (virtually none), and they were more likely than the Massachusetts sample to have incomes at least twice the poverty level.

Although more of the CCRC residents had one or more medically limiting conditions (although not significantly so in the youngest and oldest groups), they tended to have a greater ability to carry out instrumental activities of daily living (IADL) such as taking out the garbage and shopping. They also were more mobile than their age peers in the traditional community, and in the oldest groups they tended to have fewer impairments in basic activities of daily living (ADL) such as bathing and personal care. They were more likely than the traditional-community sample to name a friend as an informal helper, and, except for the youngest age category, they spent more time phoning and visiting friends and went out of the house more often. But across all age categories the Massachusetts sample spent more time visiting and phoning family, and more named a child among those who provided help or would provide help if needed.

Responses to the question of where people should live when they reach old age and are unable to care for themselves physically point to a greater predilection for an independent life style on the part of elderly people who choose CCRCs compared with their age peers in the general community. More than three quarters of CCRC residents compared with less than 40 percent in each age category said they wanted to live in their own home with help. We found glaring differences in the percentages who responded that they had never thought of it and/or did not want to think of it. Considering the long-term care planning features of a CCRC, it was not surprising that few CCRC residents gave this response (less than 4 percent in any of the age categories). In contrast, between 26 and 40 percent in the Massachusetts age groups under 85 years and almost a quarter 85 and older responded in this manner.

Extended and Limited CCRCs

The nineteen CCRCs from which the samples were drawn for these analyses were nonprofit private-sector ventures. As in the 1991 national survey of CCRCs (AAHA and Ernst and Young 1992), on average, the extended CCRCs were considerably larger than the limited CCRCs. Other than one limited CCRC that had been in operation for ninety-six years in 1986, the range in years of operation for the extended and limited CCRCs in our study was roughly similar (from two to twenty-two years). Occupancy rates of both types of CCRC were high, but the extended CCRCs had a higher mean rate of occupancy (99 percent) than did the limited CCRCs (90 percent).

Two of the nine extended CCRCs but seven of the ten limited CCRCs had personal care (assisted living) units. The ratio of nursing home beds to apartments was similar in the two types of CCRC (0.37 in extended and 0.34 in limited CCRCs). The nursing home beds in the majority of both types of facility were Medicare certified, some of which had Medicaid certification as well. Only two of the nine extended CCRCs and three of the ten limited CCRCs had neither Medicaid nor Medicare certification.

Both the extended and limited study CCRCs offered many amenities, with the limited CCRCs offering at least as many as the extended facilities. However, in addition to the added protection against high costs of nursing home care, on average, extended CCRCs included more health and supportive services — meals, light housekeeping, laundry (linens), and transportation — in the monthly fee. Correspondingly, the mean entrance and monthly fees of extended CCRCs were higher than those of limited CCRCs.

Entrance Characteristics of Residents of Extended and Limited CCRCs

For the most part, entrance characteristics of the residents of extended and limited CCRCs were similar and followed the same patterns, even when there were significant differences between the residents in the two types of facility. We found no significant differences between recent residents or between longer-stay residents in these communities in the percentages who were female, lived alone at admission to the facility, had participated in the work force for most of their lives, had visited other communities before entrance, or had owned their own home before CCRC entrance (condominiums as well as private houses, whether in age-integrated or in retirement communities).

Longer-stay residents of extended CCRCs tended to be older than those of limited CCRCs. But in both types of community, the average age at entrance seems to be increasing — the mean age of recent residents was 77.9 and 78.4 years, respectively, for extended and limited CCRC residents at admission, and for longer-stay residents, it was 76.3 and 77.1 years. Despite the older age, more couples are moving into both types of CCRC. For limited CCRCs in particular, there appears to be an expansion of interest among persons other than college graduates (38 percent of recent compared with 48 percent of longer-stay limited CCRC residents graduated from college; among extended CCRC residents, 55 percent of the recent and 61 percent of the longer-stay residents were college graduates).

In fact, the largest difference between extended and limited CCRC residents (both recent and longer stay) was in educational status. Although sizable proportions of residents in each of the samples came from a private house in an age-integrated community (regardless of whether or not they owned their homes), significantly larger proportions of recent and longer-stay residents who had entered limited (more than half) than extended CCRCs (approximately half) did so. Conversely, although only a minority in each of the groups moved to the CCRC from another retirement community (less than one quarter of the residents in the largest group), proportionately more of those moving to extended CCRCs had done so. It appears that more individuals moving into extended CCRCs had prior experience living in an age-segregated (older adult) community. (Other retirement communities that have no pooled-risk features either for nursing home care or supportive services may represent a particularly good market for organizations planning to develop extended CCRC facilities.)

Baseline Characteristics of Residents of Extended and Limited CCRCs

Although baseline was less than a year after entrance for recent residents — for many, within two weeks after entrance — for longer-stay residents it might have been years after entrance. Not only would longer-stay residents have been older, but marital status, health and functional status, and other quality-of-life characteristics might well have changed.

Residents in the two types of CCRC were similar at baseline in whether they lived alone/not alone, in three of the four marital status variables (considered separately, the percentages married, separated or divorced, and never married), and in the two residential propinquity variables (mean number of children within a one-hour drive and the mean number of relatives within a one-hour drive). Of particular note, CCRC residents in general appear to have only a small number of living children. In these samples there was an average of less than 1.4 in any of the groups. On average, one third or fewer of these children were nearby (the average was more for recent and less for longer-stay residents, but still no more than 0.49 in any of the groups). It is obvious that many CCRC residents were not in a position to call on children for informal help even if they had wanted to do so.

We found a number of differences having life style implications between residents of the two types of CCRC:

- Significantly fewer residents of extended than of limited CCRCs were widowed.
- Extended CCRC residents had fewer medical problems and tended to report better health than their counterparts in limited CCRCs (but the mean self-rated health of even these residents was in the good range).
- A higher percentage of residents of extended than of limited CCRCs drew upon interest from savings, investments, or trust funds to finance the monthly fee.
- In the month before baseline, the majority in each sample had spent

less than $100 on medical expenses, but residents of limited CCRCs had more out-of-pocket medical expenses (above and beyond what they received from Medicare and/or health insurance) than did extended CCRC residents.

▪ Aside from vacations, residents of extended CCRCs regularly spent more money for entertainment outside the home for activities such as movies, plays, concerts, and sporting events. Since there was little difference in the amenities that each type of CCRC provided, the difference in expenditures on outside entertainment may have reflected differences in economic status. It might also have been a function of life-style differences or a combination of both.

Reasons for Entering

Adding to an understanding of the kinds of persons who become CCRC residents, a major conclusion from the analyses of reasons for entrance is that elderly persons who choose a CCRC living arrangement tend to act very rationally. Their reasons for selecting their CCRC are in line with the services that it offers.

At baseline, we asked residents which of eight reasons for entering their CCRC applied to them. Except for the desire to be with people like themselves (with 39 and 43 percent, respectively, of recent and longer-stay residents claiming this reason), close to half or more of each sample said that each of the reasons probed applied to them. Access to needed services ranked very high as did guaranteed protective features of the contract, regardless of CCRC type. For recent entrants, access to needed services was the most pervasive reason. For longer-stay residents, access to needed services was also the most pervasive reason for limited CCRC residents, but guaranteed protective features were the most pervasive for residents of extended CCRCs. Cohen (1988) reported comparable findings.

Significantly more residents of limited than of extended CCRCs, regardless of length of stay, said that living close to friends/relatives or near a familiar area, desirability of apartment/location, compensating for the absence or potential absence of helpers, and wanting to be with people like themselves were among their reasons. Significantly more of the extended CCRC residents indicated that guaranteed protective features of the contract were a consideration in their choosing the CCRC. Although more so among recent than longer-stay residents in each type of CCRC, we found no difference in the percentages saying that avoiding pressure/demands on their family or friends was among their reasons for entering.

At follow-up, we asked residents which of fourteen characteristics of retirement communities they considered important (whether very or somewhat important) in their decision to move to the CCRC. The characteristics were: a nice apartment unit, extensive common areas, high-quality image and decor, location, security and safety, housekeeping services, meals available in the dining room, personal care services, nursing home available, maintenance and yard work done, system for handling medical emergencies, transportation furnished, fees included nursing home care, and guaranteed residence even if income drops.

Except for the last three reasons, the majority of both extended and limited CCRC residents thought that each of these characteristics was at least of some importance in their choice of CCRC. As might be expected, the largest difference between residents of extended and limited CCRCs was in the proportion saying that the inclusion of nursing home care in the fees was important in their decision to move in. Approximately 90 percent of recent and longer-stay residents in extended CCRCs made this claim compared with about one third of the residents in limited CCRCs. In fact, this was the reason least likely to be given by these residents. Although more than half of both recent and longer-stay residents of extended CCRCs said that furnished transportation was of some importance, it was the reason that fewest claimed to be important. Among residents of limited CCRCs, fewer than half considered it an important reason. Guaranteed residence in the face of a reduction in income was considered important by about three quarters of extended CCRC residents and roughly half of those in limited CCRCs.

Scores on scales measuring reasons for entering pointed to distinct differences between those of the extended and limited CCRC residents. Residents of extended CCRCs consistently considered health and financial concerns and IADL/environmental services more important than did residents of limited CCRCs. Residents of limited CCRCs consistently considered location to be more important than did extended CCRC residents.

Residents in the Light of Their CCRC Experience

There was a striking similarity in the pattern of responses of residents of extended and limited CCRCs regarding their use of facility amenities, participation in activities both before and after joining the CCRC, and attitudes and perceptions of the CCRC living arrangement. However, we found significant differences (often small) between residents in the two types of facility, and they were generally in favor of the residents of extended CCRCs.

Of the five resources commonly available in all nineteen of the study CCRCs, the rank order of use was identical for residents of extended and limited CCRCs, regardless of length of stay. From most to least used they were: library, chapel, crafts/activities room, game room, and health club/exercise classes. In both types of community a majority of residents used the library, but only a minority (approximately one quarter or fewer of the residents) used the health club or attended exercise classes. Differences that we observed between residents of extended and limited CCRCs in the degree of use of CCRC amenities appeared to be a function of variations in the distribution of characteristics (health, age, and related variables) of the samples rather than attributable to the facilities.

CCRC residents in both types of community generally participated in half or more of fifteen activities probed (and probably participated in other activities that we did not query). On the whole, the extended CCRC residents participated in significantly more activities than did the residents of limited CCRCs; but at least of the longer-stay residents, more of the residents of limited CCRCs participated in volunteer activities. In this case, although health and age were related to participation, differences in age and health did not account for the disparities we observed between residents of the two types of CCRC.

Although residents of both CCRC types tended to be an active population, they participated in fewer activities than they had as younger adults (before joining the CCRC). Only a small percentage of each group participated in new types of activity after joining the CCRC. Attending lectures and volunteer activities elicited the highest percentage of new participants. All the same, no more than 6 percent attended lectures, and no more than 7 percent participated in volunteer activities for the first time only after moving to the CCRC.

In general, satisfaction with the CCRC was high for all groups on all aspects probed. Furthermore, for recent and longer-stay residents in either type of CCRC, complaints about the unavailability of services when needed were conspicuous by their absence. However, sizable minorities of most of these samples responded unfavorably to two questions. At follow-up, 39 percent of the recent and 30 percent of longer-stay residents of limited CCRCs (and 22 percent of the recent and 14 percent of extended CCRC residents) responded unfavorably to the question of whether the CCRC was living up to their expectations. As many as 36 percent of the recent and 41 percent of the longer-stay residents of limited CCRCs and 34 percent of the recent and longer-stay residents of extended CCRCs said they did not have an opportunity to influence management.

Scores on two indices measuring aspects of quality of life once again attested to the similarity in the pattern of responses of residents in the two types of CCRC. One was a seven-point quality-of-life scale (including a cluster of social interaction, unmet needs, and self-reported health variables identified through factor analysis). Although the patterning of responses was similar across samples in both types of community, and we found no difference between recent residents, longer-stay extended CCRC residents tended to score better at follow-up on this quality-of-life scale than did residents of limited CCRCs. The analysis controlling for initial differences in the two populations supported this finding.

Findings for the second index, which measured attitudes toward own aging and was an identified and standardized component of the larger PGC Morale Scale (Morris and Sherwood 1975), were particularly useful for insights regarding potential benefits of the CCRC living arrangement. Although not for the longer-stay samples, significant within-sample changes from baseline to follow-up did occur for recent residents of both types of CCRC. In each case, their attitudes toward their own aging significantly improved from baseline to follow-up. Although the analysis controlling for baseline differences between these two samples indicated that residents of extended facilities were particularly better off, the improved attitude of residents in both types of community suggested that CCRCs in general provide an environment conducive to changing the picture one has of one's own aging in a positive way and that it does not take long for attitudinal improvement to occur. After a while, however, the change levels off.

Quality of Life in CCRC and Traditional-Community Populations

Combining the samples in extended and limited CCRCs, comparisons between CCRC residents age 70 and older and age peers in the Massachusetts community revealed consistent differences between the two populations on fourteen of seventeen variables measuring aspects of the quality of life. In some respects, however, the two populations experienced similar outcomes, although some of the differences in outcome at follow-up disappeared when we controlled key baseline differences in characteristics.

As might be expected, health and functional status deteriorated at least to some degree between baseline and follow-up for each of the samples as a whole. Nevertheless, even at follow-up the majority in both samples — often a large majority (80 percent or more) — enjoyed good health and reported no impairment in most of the functional status areas investigated. CCRC residents generally had higher self-reported health ratings and, on average, were more self-sufficient, had fewer ADL impairments (e.g., bathing, transfer out of a chair, personal care), had fewer IADL problems (e.g., taking out garbage, shopping, and transportation), and were more mobile. However, except for problems with IADL, follow-up differences in health and functional status disappeared when we controlled key baseline differences.

Controlled analyses also changed the follow-up findings for two variables: the number of unmet needs and the number of informal helpers who could be counted on indefinitely (as long as needed). Although at follow-up we found the Massachusetts sample to have fewer unmet needs than CCRC residents, the difference between the two samples appeared to be a function of differences in baseline characteristics. Estimates based on controlled analysis indicate that if the two samples were more alike on these characteristics (e.g., having more children nearby), CCRC residents would actually have done better. Second, although the number was less than at baseline for both samples, we found no difference at follow-up between CCRC and traditional-community residents in the number of informal helpers who could be counted on indefinitely (as long as needed). However, it appears again that had the two samples been more alike at baseline, the CCRC residents would likely have experienced less loss than the traditional-community residents in the number of informal helpers who could be relied upon indefinitely.

Controlled analyses did not change the findings for a number of follow-up outcomes. CCRC residents were more likely than the Massachusetts sample to leave the house more than once a week, to spend more time interacting (by phone or visiting) with friends, and to have enough money to live on without trouble. The Massachusetts sample was likely to spend more time visiting or phoning family, to have more informal helpers, and to have a confidante.

Comparisons of Selected Costs of Care

We adopted a Medicare-specific perspective in this aspect of the study; that is, we did not include in the analysis services not covered by Medicare and out-of-pocket expenditures for deductibles, copayments, and fees above the Medicare-designated customary, reasonable, or prevailing threshold. The medical services included inpatient hospital care, skilled nursing home care, home health care, and physician care rendered in a hospital, nursing home, or ambulatory setting. We compared costs over a one-year period.

A larger percent of the CCRC sample than of the Massachusetts group reported using one or more medical services (96 vs. 86 percent) during the twelve-month period after baseline. Among those who used any care, average annual expenditures were higher for the Massachusetts sample ($2,625 vs. $1,936), but this difference was not significant at the p 0.05 level. When we spread expenditures over the entire sample, average annual expenditures were $1,772 and $2,312, respectively, for the CCRC and Massachusetts samples, again a statistically nonsignificant difference. In both samples, inpatient hospital care accounted for approximately 70 percent of total expenditures. Very few persons in each of these samples used Medicare-covered skilled nursing home or home health care. These services combined accounted for less than 2 percent of overall annual expenditures. We noted statistically significant expenditure differences for only one of these services: skilled nursing home care. More individuals residing in CCRCs used this service than people living in the traditional-community setting (1.3 vs. 0.4 percent), and CCRC residents had higher average annual costs ($27 vs. $3). These averages reflected actual expenditures for those with care spread over the entire study sample; that is, both those who used care and those who did not. Cohen et al. (1989) also reported that CCRC residents had a greater risk of nursing home entries and repeat entries.

The CCRC residents had higher annual expenditures for physician care rendered within a nursing home setting than did the Massachusetts sample ($46 vs. $5) but lower expenditures for ambulatory physician care ($284 vs. $430). Expenditures for physician care rendered in a hospital did not differ across samples.

We conducted a separate analysis of expenditures in a person's last year of life. We based this analysis on self-report data that encompassed all nursing home care regardless of whether it was covered by Medicare or not. CCRC residents used more days of institutional (acute hospital and nursing home) care in their last year of life than did the traditional-community residents. However, their expenditures for institutional care were significantly lower than those incurred by non—CCRC residents. This finding pertained to the differential use of hospital care and nursing home care. The Massachusetts sample used more hospital care than did CCRC residents but less nursing home care. Comparable patterns emerged both for those who began the study period in a nursing home and for those who were not institutionalized twelve months before death.

Five Policy Issues

In Chapter 1 we raised five policy issues of major concern to the long-term care sector: (1) ensuring access (direct and financial) both to long-term supportive community and nursing home services when necessary; (2) ensuring access (direct and financial) to community-based social supports and adequate housing; (3) without eliminating the benefits of an informal care network, ensuring access while addressing the elderly person's need to retain locus of control; (4) integrating acute and long-term health care services; and (5) addressing society's concern with the high costs of medical care and developing cost-conscious interventions.

In the following sections we will summarize the project's findings with regard to these issues.

Ensuring Access to Supportive Community Services and Nursing Home Care

Clearly CCRCs represent one type of living arrangement which, at least conceptually, meets this goal. Among the eight reasons residents gave for entering their CCRC, access to needed services ranked very high, regardless of CCRC type. All of our study CCRCs appeared to have met this goal as far as supportive community services were concerned, although such services were not always included in the monthly fees. Residents exhibited a high degree of satisfaction with the CCRC. Very rarely did residents say that services were unavailable when they needed them. However, in the small number of cases where this was the case, it was more likely to have occurred for residents of limited than extended CCRCs.

Access to nursing home care was not examined directly, but the contracts in most of our study CCRCs guaranteed or assumed access to their nursing home or health center (and extended CCRCs provided this care with no or minimal extra cost beyond the monthly fee). Two of the ten limited CCRCs, however, had some reservations. Both were fee-for-service as far as nursing home care was concerned, and these communities accepted persons from outside the CCRC to fill their nursing home beds. Therefore, sometimes when a resident needed nursing home care, no bed was available. Under such conditions, the contract stipulated that the CCRC would help find adequate nursing home care. Anecdotal reports (in a period of between two to two and one half years) indicated that this situation did occur for two or three residents (not necessarily in our sample) in each of these facilities. We heard of no case in which this happened in any of the extended CCRCs.

Assuring financial access to nursing home care appears to have been particularly important to residents of extended CCRCs. A large majority of the extended CCRC residents reported that the inclusion of nursing home care as part of the entrance and monthly fees was very important in their decision to move to the CCRC; only a minority of the residents of limited CCRCs did so, and in fact this was a reason for entering least likely to be given by these residents. For the most part, the ability of the resident to pay for nursing home care was not a matter of much concern for this group or for the limited CCRC itself. Almost always facilities check for economic solvency before accepting an applicant into the community. Unless some catastrophe occurs, residents are likely to have sufficient funds to cover costs of either community or nursing home care. In this study very few persons had to spend down any part of the principal from their estates to cover costs of living at the CCRC; for example, only a very small proportion of residents, regardless of type of CCRC or length of stay, used principal from savings, trust funds, or proceeds from the sale of property to pay the monthly fees.

Findings from this study indicate that both types of community, in general, do provide direct and financial access to needed services and fulfill the goal of supplying access to community services and nursing home care even in the face of a catastrophic change in a resident's ability to pay the monthly fee (or the fee-for-services). As we pointed out in Chapter 2, although some residents may have left on their own because of a reversal in economic status, to our knowledge none of the study facilities asked a resident to leave for this reason. The contracts of some of these facilities stated specifically that residents would not be terminated solely because of an inability to pay their monthly fees (unless there had been deliberate divestment of funds). Some contracts imposed conditions upon the residents, for example, the resident had to apply for governmental benefits before the CCRC would subsidize his or her costs. We observed no difference in commitment to residents by type of CCRC. Although this commitment may not be as strong among future for-profit CCRCs, the security feature was apparent in currently operated CCRCs as represented by our sample. Perhaps this will become a feature that distinguishes between CCRCs and offshoots of CCRCs which provide access to services but no element of pooled risk.

We should note that we made no particular attempt to select for this study CCRCs with "better" reputations, and we believe that no systematic bias of this sort accounted for our results. For practical purposes we looked for geographic areas with relatively high concentrations of CCRCs and sought the participation of facilities that were no more than sixty to ninety minutes from the field worker in that state. For the most part before beginning the study we had no knowledge of the reputations of the CCRCs that agreed to participate.

Ensuring Access to Community-Based Social Supports and Adequate Housing

To a large extent CCRC communities, whether extended or limited, also fulfill this goal. That each of the CCRCs provided adequate housing is evidenced by the sizable majorities of residents in these facilities who said that location, having a nice apartment, high-quality image and decor, extensive common areas, and security and safety of the CCRC were at least of some importance in their choice of CCRC. Furthermore, at follow-up, very few residents (less than 5 percent) said that they were dissatisfied with their housing.

CCRCs also afford opportunities to develop social supports. As exemplified in this study, both types of CCRC offered many amenities and leisure activity programs on campus. This type of environment stimulates and provides activities and social interactions and fosters developing friendships among residents. Indirectly, at least, social relationships among residents might ultimately lead not only to social support but to mutual help of some type (e.g., performing small errands, jointly going shopping for clothing). The greater proportion of CCRC residents compared with traditional-community residents who named a friend among those considered key informal helpers supports this theory. CCRC supportive services might also free up time that the resident might otherwise spend in performing IADL (e.g., in meal preparation and housekeeping) and would leave the resident with more energy to interact with friends and to participate with others in leisure-time activities.

Project findings concerning social interactions support this hypothesis. CCRC residents spent more time phoning or visiting friends than did traditional-community residents who were at least 70 years old. In fact, we observed an increase in interaction with friends between baseline and follow-up for CCRC residents, whereas the level of interaction with friends remained the same for the Massachusetts group. Both at baseline and at follow-up, more than 90 percent of the CCRC residents said they were satisfied with the social and leisure activities available at their facility.

To some extent, the freed-up energy that facilitates higher levels of interactions with friends and other leisure activities may also affect the residents' perceptions about their health status. For example, even though they had at least as many limiting medical conditions, CCRC residents tended to perceive themselves as being in better health than did their counterparts in the traditional community.

At least one other finding points to the supportive social environment of CCRCs. Although not for the longer-stay samples, significant within-sample changes from baseline to follow-up occurred for recent residents of both types of CCRC. In each case, their attitudes toward their own aging improved significantly from baseline to follow-up. This suggests that CCRCs, regardless of type, provide an environment conducive to changing in a positive way the picture one has of one's own aging and that it does not take long for attitudinal improvement to occur (although this improvement eventually levels off).

However, the CCRC environment does not necessarily stimulate social interaction with relatives. Both at baseline and at follow-up, the Massachusetts sample spent more time visiting and talking with family members. Time spent phoning and visiting family members increased from baseline to follow-up in each of the groups, but the increase was larger for the Massachusetts sample. As we noted in Chapter 4, increased interaction with family members for both samples might be the elderly persons' response to perceived threats to their own health and physical functioning. Although by no means a total explanation, the lesser inter-action between family and residents of CCRCs may have been a function of opportunity. CCRC residents were less likely to have children, and close to three quarters compared with only a little more than one quarter of the Massachusetts sample had no children living nearby (within a one-hour drive).

Along with greater interaction with family members, proportion-ately more of the Massachusetts sample also said that there was someone that they felt particularly close to — someone with whom they could be completely themselves, and in whom they had complete trust and confi-dence (a confidante). Interactions with relatives, particularly result-ing from their response to increased supportive service needs of the el-derly people, may also enhance the feelings of confidence and trust in these family members. From this perspective, traditional-community residents have more opportunity than CCRC residents to develop inti-mate relationships.

Benefits of Informal Care and Ensuring Access while
Retaining Locus of Control

Without eliminating the benefits of an informal network, ensuring access while retaining locus of control is a complicated issue. CCRC residents certainly enjoy access to adequate housing, to community sup-port services and nursing care when needed, and to certain types of social support. Nevertheless, to the extent that increased interaction with fam-ily members is likely to strengthen emotional involvement and support, it would seem that residence in a CCRC in some respects does not neces-sarily promote benefits that may be derived when supportive services are provided by loved ones in the informal care network — children and other family members. In general, in addition to the emotional support that can be expected from interaction with family members and having a confi-dante, elderly people in the general population appear likely to have more informal helpers (almost always family members). In this study, on aver-age, the number of informal helpers decreased from baseline to follow-up for CCRC residents but increased for the Massachusetts sample. This finding persisted even when baseline differences in characteristics of these two populations were taken into consideration. To the extent that the number of informal helpers decreased more than it otherwise would have, some of the potential benefits of an informal care system may have been lost.

At follow-up, both traditional-community and CCRC residents had fewer informal helpers whom they believed could be relied upon indefinitely than they had at baseline, with a similar number of such persons reported by each of these populations. On a more positive note for the CCRC population, however, controlled analyses indicated that if the two populations had been more alike in baseline characteristics (in particular, in the number of children nearby and whether or not they lived alone), the situation would have been reversed, with the CCRC residents likely to have had a higher number of informal helpers on whom they could rely indefinitely.

Indirectly, at least, the supportive and long-term care services available at the CCRC shape the kinds of services that might be required of such informal helpers on an indefinite basis — services that are not likely to be particularly burdensome. Residents may be in a mutual-help relationship with their informal helpers. CCRC residents have no need of many of the services, such as meal preparation and housecleaning, which informal care givers of elderly traditional-community residents often provide. Moving in with the care giver is also not a concern of CCRC residents. Certainly elderly persons in the traditional community are more likely than CCRC residents to receive informal help that is vital to their remaining in their current setting. The informal care system of CCRC residents, then, could be expected to play a qualitatively different, more minor, and less burdensome role than that often played by informal care networks of elderly traditional-community residents. This in turn may lead CCRC residents to be more confident that they could count on informal helpers indefinitely.

It can also be argued that the qualitatively different role of the informal care system of CCRC residents has positive implications for the goal of empowering the elderly person to maintain a more independent life style — that is, to have access to needed services while retaining the locus of control. Having to depend upon informal care givers for basic ADL may weaken the elderly person's ability to control his or her own destiny. This may be particularly the case when the elderly person must move in with a relative. When the relative is the elderly person's child, role reversal may occur, with the child assuming the parental role.

Moving to a CCRC may also impact negatively on a person's locus of control, particularly if the CCRC operators adopt a paternalistic philosophy. Although the majority of residents believed that they had an opportunity to influence management decisions that affected them, sizable minorities in both extended and limited CCRCs disagreed. Of the areas probed, this was perhaps the greatest source of discontent, suggesting an area of concern and inquiry when choosing a CCRC.

Although only a small number of communities have marketed themselves as condominiums or cooperatives, including the concept of equity in the CCRC living arrangement may enhance the locus of control while providing the resident with access to needed services. It remains to be seen whether this type of arrangement will spread and whether the resident-owners then have more input into management.

Integrating Acute and Long-Term Health Care Services

Except for general questions about satisfaction with services and satisfaction with the CCRC, interviews with residents did not address the integration of acute and long-term health care services. Nevertheless, the high level of satisfaction of these residents, along with organizational data gathered about the study CCRCs, and the concepts underlying the CCRC movement suggest that CCRCs are successful in fulfilling this goal. Reports by other researchers also support this conclusion (Bishop 1988; Newcomer and Preston 1994).

A continuum-of-care perspective, in which residential care and nursing care are provided as needed, coordinated or managed by the administrator, is an underlying characteristic of CCRCs. In the opinion of some analysts, CCRCs represent a form of managed care for the long-term care sector (Cohen et al. 1989; Somers and Livengood 1992) and a care delivery system that may also actively embody a concept of health promotion (Somers and Spears 1992).

For residents transferred permanently to a facility's nursing home, the CCRC takes on direct responsibility for coordination of care, including decisions about treating acute care conditions in the nursing home itself, when to hospitalize the nursing home resident, and about continued care after hospitalization. In our study at least indirectly the recognition of the need to coordinate acute care and long-term care services was evident in the contract references to temporary care that might be needed in the CCRC nursing home, for example, for recuperative care after hospitalization.

Management of residential care in the ILUs also necessitates consideration of acute health care needs. Even without systemized procedures to do so, CCRC managers are likely to gain knowledge of serious acute conditions, particularly when a resident is unable to attend meals. Obviously facilities routinely make some adjustments in response to supportive care needs associated with acute and long-term conditions (e.g., tray service for persons temporarily confined to bed, special diets). Going a step further, some communities (more so among the extended CCRCs in our study) take a more direct responsibility for managing health care, sometimes as part of the monthly fee (usually requiring that the resident purchase health insurance policies, including all public forms of health insurance for which they are eligible). In our study a number of the extended CCRCs covered prescription medicines, physician services, and hospitalization, including medical and surgical services, as part of the monthly fee (although coverage was limited to services provided by medical and nursing staff affiliated with, or referred by, the CCRC). All of the extended CCRCs recognized that transitions were sometimes needed and offered temporary nursing care in a skilled nursing unit at no more than the charge for extra meals served in the nursing facility. Most of the limited CCRCs also offered temporary nursing home care (for a limited number of days), charging on a discounted basis or only for the extra meals.

Societal Concern with High Costs of Medical Care

CCRCs, particularly extended CCRCs, attempt to address this issue, at least from the point of view of the elderly consumer. As indicated, for many residents inclusion of supportive services and nursing home care in the entrance and monthly fees was a motivating force in the decision to join the CCRC. Communities that clearly operate on a pooled-risk model can be considered a type of cost-conscious intervention (in particular, extended CCRCs and those limited CCRCs that provide substantial discounts or charge a relatively small part of the actual costs of care in the facility's nursing home).

CCRCs that include almost all or a large percentage of the costs of nursing home care as part of the entrance and monthly fees need to manage resident care to avoid the likelihood of permanent institutionalization. To the extent that these communities also assume responsibility for a broad spectrum of health care services as part of the monthly fee, the high costs of medical care become a prime concern. In our study, the CCRCs providing the most extensive health coverage usually required residents to purchase long-term care and other health insurance policies, including all public forms of health insurance for which they were eligible. For residents and/or the CCRCs, Medicare benefits might help defray the costs of temporary placement for rehabilitative care in the facility's nursing home after hospitalization (e.g., after a hip fracture or a stroke).

Some CCRCs do not want to be involved in third-party payments and either cover long-term care totally as part of the entrance or monthly fees or, in limited CCRCs, expect direct payment from the resident for nursing home care. If care in the nursing home shortens acute hospital stays or if Medicare benefits are not used to pay for physician services and nursing care provided by the CCRC, public costs are likely to be less. But it is also possible that CCRCs will encourage residents to make greater use of resources that are covered by public forms of health insurance.

Shedding some light on this subject, in this study we adopted a Medicare-specific perspective in the comparative analyses of costs of care. We included only services covered by Medicare, not out-of-pocket expenditures for deductibles, copayments, and fees above the Medicare designated customary, reasonable, or prevailing threshold.

As indicated previously by the cost analysis, although the large majority in both populations used medical services, a larger percent of the CCRC group than of the Massachusetts sample reported using one or more medical services. However, average annual expenditures were not higher for CCRC residents. Actually, the average annual expenditures were higher for the Massachusetts population, but the difference was not statistically significant.

In both samples, inpatient hospital care accounted for about 70 percent of total expenditures, with only a few persons using Medicare-covered skilled nursing home or home health care (accounting for less than 2 percent of the Medicare-covered expenditures). Nonetheless, CCRC residents spent more time in skilled nursing homes, resulting in higher average annual costs for this service. Cohen et al. (1989) also reported that CCRC residents had a greater risk of nursing home entry and repeat entries.

Although CCRC residents had higher annual expenditures than traditional-community residents for physician care rendered within a nursing home setting, they had lower expenditures for ambulatory physician care. We found no difference between these samples for hospital-stay physician care.

The separate analysis on expenditures in a person's last year of life, however, suggested that during this period of time, the CCRC living arrangement might have reduced costs. This analysis was based on self-report data that encompassed all nursing home care whether or not it was covered by Medicare. Costs of hospital and/or nursing home care during the last year of life were significantly lower for CCRC residents than for the Massachusetts sample. This finding results from the different way in which these groups used hospital and nursing home care:

the traditional-community residents used more hospital care than CCRC residents but less nursing home care.

Replicating the earlier work of Lubitz and Prihoda (1984), McCall (1984), and Riley et al. (1987), Lubitz and Riley (1993) confirmed the high cost of medical care which decedents incur in their last year of life. These authors suggested that the factors contributing to these high costs were inflation, new techniques, and greater intensity of care — factors that appear to call for a managed care approach.

Clearly, these findings are provocative but limited. Although it appears that substantial cost containment and savings in Medicare expenditures are likely during the last year of life, these analyses shed no light on other costs (including other public entitlements, such as Medicaid). In delving into the cost analysis more deeply, researchers should adopt a societal perspective; that is, they should include all services, whether or not covered by Medicare, and recognize all costs covered by Medicaid, Medicare supplementary policies, other health insurance, and by the person (as out-of-pocket payments).

We also have no evidence of service reduction or quality of care in relation to comparative costs of care of CCRC and traditional-community residents during their last year of life. In fact, the interrelationships among service reduction, quality of care, and comparative costs are needed areas of study. This is an issue relevant not only for the last year of life but for health care at any point in time.

Final Thoughts

From the above discussion, it can be seen that CCRCs do address the service needs and quality of life of their residents, and in one way or another this type of living arrangement touches upon each of the five policy issues raised. Conceptually and in practice, CCRCs ensure direct and financial access to supportive ADL and IADL community services and nursing home care. However, the residents must be sufficiently solvent to afford the entry fee (often substantial) and the monthly fees.

This type of living arrangement also ensures access to adequate housing and community-based social supports from friends, in particular. It seems likely that benefits of the type of help that can be expected from friends are readily gained in this type of environment, including the development of mutual help, most likely in performing small errands and shopping. But this type of setting does not necessarily lend itself to the kinds of benefits that might be derived when help with ADL and IADL is provided by children or other close relatives. At the same time, the burden on family members is less, and this in some ways may promote more positive social interactions between them and their family members and foster the residents' ability to maintain the locus of control. Furthermore, for the majority of CCRC residents, avoiding dependence on their informal network for ADL and IADL supportive services was a prime motivation for joining the CCRC and enhanced their retaining the locus of control. What is lost in one respect may be gained in other ways.

Since an underlying characteristic of CCRCs is the coordination and management of residential and nursing home care, it can be expected that, to some degree, integration of acute and long-term needs of residents occurred — at least a rudimentary form of managed care. The issue of the role of CCRCs in assuring continuity of care and its relation to managed care is certainly an intriguing one. It is an important area of needed comparative research both now and in the future as alternate models of managed care are developed.

Currently there is variation in the extent to which these communities practice managed care, with some providing extensive services. Of the nineteen study CCRCs, extended CCRCs appear more likely to practice a more advanced form of this service. The contracts of five of the nine communities referred to a broad range of community health services in addition to long-term care in the nursing home. Although coverage was limited to services provided by medical and nursing staff affiliated with, or referred by, the CCRC, it included acute hospitalization, medical and surgical services, physician services, and temporary nursing care in a skilled nursing unit.

Contracts in these CCRCs, however, required that the resident purchase all public forms of health insurance for which they were eligible, and, for their residents in ILUs, it may take a long time (if ever) before public cost savings may occur, even with managed care in place. Data from the cost analyses suggest that during the last year of life, CCRCs may be a cost-containment intervention as far as Medicare costs are concerned, primarily because of the greater use of the nursing home rather than acute hospital care. Medicare-covered home health care and skilled nursing home care, areas of potential savings of public costs, accounted for less than 2 percent of the Medicare-covered expenditures. It is, of course, possible that the nursing home benefits of CCRCs may reduce public expenditures in the long run. Although greater temporary use of skilled nursing homes by CCRC residents may engender more public costs, Medicare savings might accumulate if CCRC residents use the nursing home on a temporary basis rather than acute emergency room hospitalization for flare-ups of chronic conditions. Furthermore, in extended and also in those limited CCRCs that charge much less than the market rate for nursing home care, persons who are transferred permanently to the nursing home generally will not find it necessary to exhaust their assets and become Medicaid recipients.

We should note one other consideration that has implications for costs in the long run: the possible role of CCRCs as an agent of prevention of morbid conditions. In this final section of the book, we present some thoughts about protecting the interests of CCRC residents and some comments about the future directions of CCRCs.

CCRCs as an Agent of Prevention

In the discussion concerning the integration of acute and long-term health care services, we pointed out that, in the opinion of some analysts, the community care delivery systems of CCRCs may actively embody a concept of health promotion. From this point of view, CCRCs have the potential for being a significant agent of prevention. Somers and Spears (1992) noted that some CCRCs have adopted a new emphasis on prevention as the primary focus of their health care delivery philosophy. In some respects, this represents a novel perspective, as by and large American culture still embodies pessimistic assumptions about aging (Institute of Medicine 1990). It is frequently assumed that growing old is associated with irreversible sickness and loss of vitality. A consensus is now slowly emerging that there is sufficient evidence on the benefits of health promotion and disease prevention among older adults to focus on such issues in providing care to this population group (German and Fried 1989; Institute of Medicine 1990; Kane et al. 1985; Lavizzo-Mourey and Diserens 1992; U.S. Congress Office of Technology 1985; U.S. DHHS 1991).

Lavizzo-Mourey and Diserens (1992) summarized succinctly the need to modify behaviors of older adults to reduce the risk of an adverse health event. Palmore (1970), in a study going back a quarter of a century, noted that health practices of exercise, weight control, and avoiding cigarettes were followed by less illness as measured by bed days, physician visits, hospitalization, and overall self-assessed health. Nearly a decade later Stenback et al. (1978) noted that physical inactivity, smoking, and immoderate use of alcohol were negatively related to health. Similarly, results emanating from a long-term community-based study of adult residents of Alameda County, California, which encompassed 120,000 person-years of follow-up on 7,000 people, indicated significant reduction in mortality and morbidity among elderly persons exposed to smoking cessation, physical activity, and weight control programs (Kaplan and Haan 1989; Wingard et al. 1982).

There has been extensive additional evidence for specific health enhancement programs. Among older adults health improvements have resulted from earlier disease detection. Morrison et al. (1988) and Shapiro et al. (1985) presented such evidence for breast cancer screening; Muller et al. (1990) reported on the benefit of screening for cervical cancer; and Ransohoff and Lang (1993) and Selby (1993) provided strong support for the need for colorectal screening among the elderly population. Researchers have also demonstrated convincingly the gains derived from hypertension detection and control (Hypertension Detection and Follow-up Program 1977; Leaverton et al. 1990; SHEP 1991; VA Cooperative Study 1970; White et al. 1990).

Many distinct preventive initiatives are possible, some of which are already in place. Many CCRCs have health clinics and screen for a number of conditions. Even if they are not currently set up for this purpose, the facilities of the CCRC nursing home often can be. Many if not most of the CCRCs currently in operation already sponsor exercise programs or health clubs; this was a common feature in all nineteen of the study CCRCs. At the same time we should note that of five resources available in all nineteen facilities, health clubs and exercise classes were least likely to be used — only a minority (between 20 and 26 percent of the recent and 19 percent of the longer-stay residents) said that they went to the health club or attended exercise classes. This percentage may be large considering the age group as a whole, but, given the potential benefits of this type of resource, it would seem that a concerted effort by CCRC operators to increase participation might be in order. To the extent that CCRCs adopt preventive initiatives (including screening and the promotion of exercise programs/health clubs), we may find beneficial outcomes with respect to utilization, cost, and quality of life.

Protecting the Interests of CCRC Residents

Although not a focus of this study, there are reasons to be concerned about ensuring that CCRCs provide appropriate care (U.S. Senate 1983) and safeguarding the residents' investment (entry fee) (Ruchlin 1987; Topolnicki 1985). Even though the occurrence of major problems may be rare, advocates of regulation point to experience with the nursing home industry as an indication that the marketplace is an inadequate mechanism for protecting residents' interests (Cohen 1980).

At present the federal government has little role in regulating CCRCs other than requiring that those seeking Medicare and/or Medicaid certification for their nursing home beds meet federal standards. But some CCRCs do not want to be involved in third-party payments. Of the nineteen study CCRCs, five had neither Medicare nor Medicaid certification.

To the extent that regulation exists, it has been left to the states. In 1991, thirty-five states had statutes regarding CCRCs; but, even aside from differences in the agencies assigned oversight and their problems in implementing the regulations, there is little uniformity across these states in definitions, certification requirements, mandatory content of contracts, provisions for escrow of entry fees, reserve fund requirements, and the like (Netting and Wilson 1994).

Recognizing the contribution to establishing and maintaining standards of care which accreditation by professional organizations has made, in 1986 the AAHA sponsored an independent national accrediting commission for CCRCs, the Continuing Care Accreditation Commission (CCAC). This commission is responsible for setting standards, accrediting, and then monitoring accredited retirement communities. This assures residents and potential entrants that the CCRC meets the criteria for sound financial operations, governance and administration, disclosure, resident life, and quality health care. Even though application for accreditation is voluntary, the CCAC accreditation program can be used by states as either a component of or a substitute for state regulations (Continuing Care Accreditation Commission 1987). By midsummer 1988, 46 CCRCs in fifteen states had been accredited; by midsummer 1995, the program had quadrupled—180 CCRCs in twenty-nine states had already been accredited, and 29 CCRCs in ten states were scheduled for review.

Other professional organizations are also interested in helping to develop standards and methods to assess CCRCs; for example, the American Academy of Actuaries and the CCAC have worked together to further this end (Sherwood et al. 1989). Working to refine the criteria of acceptability and develop effective assessment tools with other interested professional organizations on an ongoing basis can inform, help test, as well as enrich the CCAC accreditation process and make it more meaningful, flexible, and responsive in fulfilling its goals. Such cooperative efforts can result in updated information for potential consumers and CCRC operators in maintaining fiscal responsibility and high standards of care.

In the long run, the CCAC accreditation program may in fact be an effective mechanism for safeguarding residents' investment and ensuring appropriate high-quality care. However, even if it proves to be an effective mechanism for residents of CCRCs that apply for certification, accreditation by the CCAC is by no means a universal requirement for operating a CCRC. Concern remains that some form of protection may be needed both for residents of CCRCs that are not interested in applying for accreditation and for residents of CCRCs that have been denied accreditation.

Future Directions

A final comment is warranted about the direction of future entry-fee CCRCs. To the extent that the large-scale surveys conducted by AAHA and Ernst and Young are representative of the field, although for-profit corporations have entered the field, the overwhelming proportion of CCRCs are nonprofit and are likely to remain so for the foreseeable future. Furthermore, the overall trend of the industry as a whole is clearly toward extended agreements (AAHA and Ernst and Young 1992). In 1988, 36 percent of CCRCs in the National Continuing Care Data Base were what has been defined as extended CCRCs, and in 1990 there were as many as 43 percent, with a reduction of from 38 percent in 1988 to 28 percent in 1990 of fee-for-service CCRCs (as opposed to limited facilities offering some long-term care benefits within the monthly fee structure). Of new communities opening from 1986 to 1991, 63 percent were extended CCRCs. This was the case even though CCRCs with limited contracts assume less risk for the medical care of their residents. There is evidence of an inverse relationship between the extent of nursing care provided and a facility's financial viability (Ruchlin 1988).

Recently, some facilities have developed a mix of contracts (extended and limited) among which prospective applicants can choose. Why a CCRC would offer a mix of contracts needs to be explored; most likely it is to make the community more financially sound and, particularly for CCRCs with empty apartments, more appealing to prospective applicants. Anecdotally, for example, it has been reported that CCRCs have difficulty in filling studio apartments whereas in the same CCRC, applicants for one- and two-bedroom apartments may have to wait for several years before one becomes available. Such facilities may be seeking ways of raising their occupancy levels by offering more than one option. Whether this strategy is successful in raising the occupancy level, and the ways in which, if any, this strategy impacts the level of satisfaction of the CCRC residents need to be explored.

The growth of rentals offering similar services without requiring an entry fee may also be reducing interest in fee-for-service CCRCs, even though these rentals (often for-profit enterprises) do not generally *guarantee* access to nursing home care and are not committed to retaining in the community residents who are experiencing economic hardships. Rather than CCRCs, such rentals may very well appeal to elderly people who are not themselves committed to remaining in the same community, who are not particularly concerned with the issue of access or planning for access when needed, and who may want to be in control of choice of care now and in the future, including the choice of long-term care facility when such services are needed.

Nevertheless, CCRCs steadily continue to be a growth industry (AAHA and Ernst and Young 1992). It is likely that extended and limited facilities with reputations for good health care and which offer at least some financial benefits when nursing home care is needed will continue to thrive in the foreseeable future. They will be particularly interesting to persons who are both concerned with access to high-quality long-term care when needed and want to ensure that their financial status will not be seriously compromised should extended nursing home care be necessary.

Many of the advantages of living in a CCRC apply equally to both limited and extended CCRCs. CCRCs to some extent can be considered a form of managed long-term care. Data from this study suggest that extended CCRCs may be particularly likely to develop and implement an even broader managed care approach. But residential and nursing care in one location, coordinated or managed by the administrator, is a fundamental characteristic of both limited or extended CCRCs. The current interest in managed care in the acute care sector of the health care field could easily spill over into the long-term care sector. If it does, CCRCs appear to deserve serious consideration as a quality-enhancing and potentially cost-effective way to institute the managed care concept into the long-term care system.

However, an important caveat must be recognized. As currently structured, CCRCs are viable options primarily for the wealthier segments of society. In some rare instances HUD[1] has subsidized nonprofit communities having many of the key elements of extended CCRCs: there is an understanding that the elderly person can ordinarily expect to remain in the community for the rest of his or her life, and the community has a continuum of living arrangements (apartments, personal care units, and nursing home beds) in one location coordinated or managed by the administrator, with the residents moving from their apartments to more dependent living arrangements when they become debilitated and need such care. However, given fiscal restraints and the funding climate during the 1990s, it is unlikely that we will see a substantial expansion of HUD-subsidized communities for some time to come. Planning efforts and new financial sources would be needed to put CCRCs within the reach of the rest of the population.

1. U.S. Department of Housing and Urban Development.

APPENDIX A

Economic and Poverty Level
Data Sources and Algorithms

In various comparisons of demographic characteristics of CCRC subsamples presented in this chapter, we derived data regarding income and poverty level from a number of sources, depending upon the particular years and age group, and population compared. We abstracted national and state population poverty level information from the literature. Because data regarding the income of CCRC sample members as well as the Massachusetts sample were not exact but rather in income categories that cut across poverty levels, we devised algorithms to classify sample members for an approximation of the proportions within these samples. Since the income cutoff for classifying persons as below or above the poverty level changes from year to year and varies by age of householder and household size, we took into consideration data for years corresponding to the date of interview.

Data Sources

Data sources for the relevant comparisons were as follows:

- National and state 1980 census data pertaining to persons 75 years and older were excerpted from the monograph by Charles F. Longino, Jr., *The Oldest Americans: State Profiles for Data Based Planning* (Coral Gables, Fla.: Center for Social Research in Aging, University of Miami, 1986).
- U.S. 1984 income and poverty level data regarding persons 65 years of age and older were derived from SSA publication 13-11871. Social Security Administration Office of Policy, Office of Research, Statistics, and International Policy, *Income of the Population 55 and Over, 1984* (Washington, D.C.: GPO, 1985), Tables 10 and 51.
- Information pertaining to income for the CCRC sample was obtained from post-test interviews with the CCRC sample, which took place between 1987 and 1988. (Note: It was not feasible to use baseline interviews since the lowest economic category referred to in the CCRC baseline interview was "Below $20,000.")
- Information pertaining to income for the Massachusetts sample was

obtained from interviews (considered baseline data in this study) with a representative sample of Massachusetts elderly persons, which were conducted as part of another study of the Department of Social Gerontological Research of the Hebrew Rehabilitation Center for Aged (Boston) during 1986 and 1987.

▪ As suggested in the *Federal Register*, vol. 55, no. 33, February 16, 1990, the Office of the Chief, Poverty and Wealth Statistics Branch, U.S. Bureau of the Census was contacted as a mechanism for obtaining precise information pertaining to federally established poverty level thresholds in 1986, 1987, and 1988 for single persons and couples 65 years of age and older (data necessary in algorithm calculations for classifying CCRC and Massachusetts comparison samples). This office provided the requested information, giving as an additional reference the *Social Security Bulletin, Annual Supplement* (1989), 123.

Algorithm for Calculating Poverty Levels for CCRC Samples Based on Data from Post-Test Interviews and Assuming That Incomes Are Distributed Equally within an Income Category

Percentage below Poverty Level

▪ *Single persons interviewed in 1987 (poverty level = $5,447):* N below poverty level = all (the N) below $5,000 plus 17.88 percent of persons with incomes between $5,000 and $7,500.
▪ *Couples interviewed in 1987 (poverty level = $6,872):* N below poverty level = all (the N) who did not live alone and who had household incomes below $5,000 plus 74.88 percent of persons with household incomes between $5,000 and $7,500.
▪ *Single persons interviewed in 1988 (poverty level = $5,674):* N below poverty level = all (the N) below $5,000 plus 26.96 percent of persons with incomes between $5,000 and $7,500.
▪ *Couples interviewed in 1988 (poverty level = $7,158):* N below poverty level = all (the N) who did not live alone and who had household incomes below $5,000 plus 86.32 percent of persons with household incomes between $5,000 and $7,500.

Add below-poverty-level Ns and divide by the total N with information for percentage below the poverty level.

Percentage Twice the Poverty Level

▪ *Single persons interviewed in 1986 (2 × poverty level = $10,450):* all (the N) above $15,000 plus 91.02 percent of persons with incomes between $10,001 and $15,000.

- *Couples interviewed in 1986 (2 × poverty level = $13,260):* all (the N) who did not live alone and who had household incomes above $15,000 plus 34.8 percent with incomes between $10,001 and $15,000.
- *Single persons interviewed in 1987 (2 × poverty level = $10,894):* all (the N) above $15,000 plus 82.12 percent of persons with incomes between $10,001 and $15,000.
- *Couples interviewed in 1987 (2 × poverty level = $13,744:* all (the N) who did not live alone and who had household incomes above $15,000 plus 25.12 percent of persons with incomes between $10,001 and $15,000.
- *Single persons interviewed in 1988 (2 × poverty level = $11,348):* all (the N) above $15,000 plus 73.04 percent of persons with incomes between $10,001 and $15,000.
- *Couples interviewed in 1988 (2 × poverty level = $14,316):* All (the N) who did not live alone and who had household incomes above $15,000 plus 13.68 percent with incomes between $10,001 and $15,000.

Add twice-poverty-level Ns and divide by total N with information for percentage twice the poverty level.

Algorithm for Calculating Poverty Levels for Massachusetts Elderly Sample Based on Data from Baseline Interviews and Assuming That Incomes Are Distributed Equally within an Income Category
Percentage below Poverty Level

- *Single persons interviewed in 1986 (poverty level = $5,225):* N below poverty level = all (the N) below $5,000 plus 10.2 percent of persons with incomes between $5,000 and $7,500.
- *Couples interviewed in 1986 (poverty level = $6,630):* N below poverty level = all (the N) who did not live alone and who had household incomes below $5,000 plus 65.2 percent of persons with household incomes between $5,000 and $7,500.
- *Single persons interviewed in 1987 (poverty level = $5,447):* N below poverty level = all (the N) below $5,000 plus 17.88 percent of persons with incomes between $5,000 and $7,500.
- *Couples interviewed in 1987 (poverty level = $6,872):* N below poverty level = all (the N) who did not live alone and who had household incomes below $5,000 plus 74.88 percent of persons with household incomes between $5,000 and $7,500.

Add below-poverty-level *N*s and divide by total *N* with information for percentage below the poverty level.

Percentage Twice the Poverty Level

- *Single persons interviewed in 1986 (2 × poverty level = $10,450):* all (the *N*) above $15,000 plus 91.02 percent of persons with incomes between $10,001 and $15,000.
- *Couples interviewed in 1986 (2 × poverty level = $13,260):* all (the *N*) who did not live alone and who had household incomes above $15,000 plus 34.8 percent with incomes between $10,001 and $15,000.
- *Single persons interviewed in 1987 (2 × poverty level = $10,894):* all (the *N*) above $15,000 plus 82.12 percent of persons with incomes between $10,001 and $15,000.
- *Couples interviewed in 1987 (2 × poverty level = $13,744:* all (the *N*) who did not live alone and who had household incomes above $15,000 plus 25.12 percent of persons with incomes between $10,001 and $15,000.

Add twice-poverty-level *N*s and divide by total *N* with information for percentage twice the poverty level.

Tables

Table B1. Standardized canonical coefficients of final discriminant functions differentiating between residents of extended and limited type CCRC

Variable	Standardized canonical coefficients	
	Recent CCRC residents	Longer-stay residents
Mean education	−0.532	−0.221
Protestant	0.144	0.347
Learned about CCRC from informal sources	0.303	−0.146
Visited other CCRCs before entrance	0.159	0.160
Home ownership before entrance	0.227	0.210
Lived in a retirement community before entrance	−0.300	−0.434
Had income from investments	0.228	0.174
No. of living children	−0.193	0.210
Financed monthly fee through:		
Interest from savings, investments, and/or trust funds	0.509	0.272
Principal from savings, trust funds, and/or proceeds from sale of property	0.362	0.154
Out-of-pocket medical expenses last month	0.271	0.357
Regularly spends money on outside entertainment	0.509	0.433
Self-sufficiency index	−0.123	0.569
Income	—[a]	−0.401
IADL index	—[a]	−0.544

[a]Although all fifteen variables were included in the analysis, income as well as IADL did not enter the final discriminant function equation for recent CCRC residents.

Table B2. Use of CCRC amenities score by self-reported health and type of CCRC

	Recent residents					
	Extended CCRC		Limited CCRC		Total	
Health rating	N	Mean	N	Mean	N	Mean
Excellent	96	2.00	45	2.11	141	2.04
Good	142	2.33	124	1.95	266	2.15
Fair/poor	43	1.56	51	1.43	94	1.49
Total	281	2.10	220	1.86	501	2.00

F tests for statistical significance of effects (two-way ANOVA)

Effect	F	p
Self-health rating	8.98	<0.001
Type of CCRC	3.11	0.078
Health rating by type of CCRC	1.61	0.202

	Longer-stay residents					
	Extended CCRC		Limited CCRC		Total	
Health rating	N	Mean	N	Mean	N	Mean
Excellent	137	2.19	121	2.40	258	2.29
Good	306	2.27	316	2.09	618	2.18
Fair/poor	109	2.06	141	1.84	250	1.94
Total	548	2.21	578	2.09	1126	2.15

F tests for statistical significance of effects (two-way ANOVA)

Effect	F	p
Self-health rating	5.31	0.005
Type of CCRC	1.83	0.176
Health rating by type of CCRC	2.76	0.064

Table B3. Use of CCRC amenities (average no. of amenities used) by age and type of CCRC

Recent residents

Age	Extended CCRC		Limited CCRC		Total	
	N	Mean	N	Mean	N	Mean
Under 75	80	2.29	54	2.37	134	2.32
75 to 85	166	2.08	123	1.72	289	1.93
85 or older	35	1.74	43	1.65	78	1.69
Total	281	2.10	220	1.86	501	2.00

F tests for statistical significance of effects

Effect	F	p
Age	6.39	0.002
Type of CCRC	3.16	0.076
Age by type of CCRC	1.47	0.232

Longer-stay residents

Age	Extended CCRC		Limited CCRC		Total	
	N	Mean	N	Mean	N	Mean
Under 75	52	2.17	39	2.03	91	2.11
75 to 85	314	2.33	307	2.21	621	2.27
85 or older	183	2.01	232	1.95	415	1.98
Total	549	2.21	578	2.10	1127	2.15

F tests for statistical significance of effects

Effect	F	p
Age	7.04	0.001
Type of CCRC	1.82	0.178
Age by type of CCRC	0.077	0.926

Note. Score = no. of five amenities; 0 = none.

Table B4. Participation in activities scales by length of residence and type of CCRC

	Recent residents							
	Extended CCRC			Limited CCRC				
	N	Mean	S.D.	N	Mean	S.D.	t	p
Participation at CCRC	281	8.01	3.12	220	7.15	3.38	2.94	0.003
Only participated before	281	3.17	2.53	220	3.22	2.74	−0.20	0.839
Never participated	281	3.59	2.30	220	4.30	2.40	3.33	0.001

	Longer-stay residents							
	Extended CCRC			Limited CCRC				
	N	Mean	S.D.	N	Mean	S.D.	t	p
Participation at CCRC	549	7.77	2.80	579	7.29	3.39	2.57	0.010
Only participated before	549	3.32	2.50	579	3.75	2.66	−2.79	0.005
Never participated	549	3.49	1.90	579	3.47	2.28	0.15	0.882

Table B5. Mean no. of activities participated in while residents of
CCRC by perceived health and type of CCRC

	Recent residents					
	Extended CCRC		Limited CCRC		Total	
Health	N	Mean	N	Mean	N	Mean
Excellent	96	8.78	45	8.36	141	8.65
Good	142	7.96	124	7.31	266	7.66
Fair/poor	43	6.47	51	5.67	94	6.03
Total	281	8.01	220	7.15	501	7.63

Effect	F	p
Self-health rating	16.90	<0.001
Type of CCRC	4.63	0.032
Health rating by type of CCRC	0.098	0.907

	Longer-stay residents					
	Extended CCRC		Limited CCRC		Total	
Health	N	Mean	N	Mean	N	Mean
Excellent	137	8.50	121	8.33	258	8.42
Good	306	7.90	316	7.48	618	7.69
Fair/poor	109	6.45	141	5.96	250	6.18
Total	548	7.76	578	7.29	1126	7.52

Effect	F	p
Self-health rating	35.64	0.001
Type of CCRC	4.40	0.036
Health rating by type of CCRC	0.22	0.806

Table B6. Mean no. of activities participated in while residents of CCRC by age and type of CCRC

	Recent residents					
	Extended CCRC		Limited CCRC		Total	
Age	N	Mean	N	Mean	N	Mean
Under 75	80	9.30	54	8.70	134	9.06
75 to 85	166	7.75	123	6.76	289	7.33
85 or older	35	6.31	43	6.30	78	6.31
Total	281	8.01	220	715	501	7.63

F tests for statistical significance of effects		
Effect	F	p
Age	20.77	<0.001
Type of CCRC	6.71	0.001
Age by type of CCRC	0.79	0.455

	Longer-stay residents					
	Extended CCRC		Limited CCRC		Total	
Age	N	Mean	N	Mean	N	Mean
Under 75	52	8.71	39	8.90	91	8.79
75 to 85	314	8.05	307	7.76	621	7.90
85 or older	183	7.01	232	6.43	415	6.69
Total	549	7.77	578	7.30	1,127	7.53

F tests for statistical significance of effects		
Effect	F	p
Age	27.19	<0.001
Type of CCRC	3.87	0.049
Age by type of CCRC	0.67	0.512

Table B7. Comparisons at follow-up

Satisfaction by length of residence and type of CCRC								
Length of residence	Extended CCRC			Limited CCRC			t	p
	N	Mean	S.D.	N	Mean	S.D.		
Less than 1 year	281	5.20	1.03	220	4.77	1.44	3.72	<0.001
1 year or more	543	5.37	1.04	579	4.75	1.44	8.27	<0.001
1 to 3 years	197	5.35	1.02	158	4.70	1.38	4.96	<0.001
3 to 6 years	156	5.25	1.15	198	4.49	1.55	5.29	<0.001
6 years or more	190	5.49	0.99	223	5.01	1.34	3.96	<0.001

No. of complaints by length of residence and type of CCRC								
Length of residence	Extended CCRC			Limited CCRC			t	p
	N	Mean	S.D.	N	Mean	S.D.		
Less than 1 year	281	0.35	0.81	220	0.60	1.32	−2.44	0.015
1 year or more	549	0.25	0.79	579	0.62	1.25	−6.04	<0.001
1 to 3 years	197	0.22	0.81	158	0.65	1.32	−3.59	<0.001
3 to 6 years	156	0.37	0.93	198	0.80	1.44	−3.37	0.001
6 years or more	190	0.17	0.63	223	0.44	0.97	−3.34	0.001

Table B8. Baseline and follow-up comparisons for CCRC and Massachusetts (MA) elderly samples: t-test was used for extended vs. limited comparisons; paired t-test was used for baseline to follow-up comparisons.

	Baseline means			Follow-up means			Baseline to follow-up means	
	CCRC (N 1,570)	MA elders (N = 1,266)	Significance	CCRC (N 1,570)	MA elders (N = 1,266)	Significance	CCRC (N = 1,570)	MA elders (N = 1,266)
Health variables								
How would you rate your health? [(1) Excellent . . . (4) Poor]	1.971	2.104	***	2.142	2.244	***	***	***
How would you describe your pain? [(1) No pain . . . (5) Horrible or excruciating]	1.577	1.661	*	1.639	1.781	***	*	***
How much of the time does bad health, sickness, or pain stop you from doing things you would like to be doing? [(1) Seldom, sometimes or never; (2) Frequently, or most of the time]	1.107	1.171	***	1.154	1.195	**	***	*
Functional health variables								
Level of self-sufficiency[a] [(1) Self-sufficient . . . (4) Most severe]	1.380	1.535	***	1.525	1.722	***	***	***
ADL impairment index[b] [(0) No impairments . . . (5) Most impairments]	0.140	0.211	**	0.308	0.428	**	***	***
IADL impairment index[c] [(0) No impairments . . . (7) Most impairments]	1.079	1.314	***	1.412	1.803	***	***	***
Mobility impairment scale[d] [(0) No impairments . . . (6) Most impairments]	0.364	0.582	***	0.691	0.826	**	***	***

Mental status

Orientation to time and place[e] [(o) No incorrect responses . . . (3) 3 Incorrect responses]

Activities/social interaction

Do you usually go out of the house (or building in which you live) more than one day a week? [(1) Yes; (2) No]

During the past week, how much time did you spend chatting on the phone or visiting in person with friends? [(1) None . . . (4) Considerable]

During the past week, how much time did you spend chatting on the phone or visiting in person with your family? [(1) None . . . (4) Considerable]

Is there anybody you feel particularly close to, that is, somebody you can be completely yourself with, and in whom you have complete trust and confidence (a confidante)? [(1) Yes; (2) No]

Informal support/inner resource

No. of informal helpers providing or currently could be relied upon for help if needed/ [(o) None . . . (4) Four helpers]

No. of informal helpers who could be relied on indefinitely (as long as needed) [(o) None . . . (4) Four helpers]

When you have to make a decision about something, in general, do you make it by yourself or do you depend upon others to make it for you? [(1) Usually by myself or with spouse; (2) Usually dependent on others]

Item								
Orientation to time and place	0.051	0.036	N.S.	0.102	0.091	N.S.	***	***
Do you usually go out of the house	1.036	1.093	***	1.027	1.143	***	N.S.	***
During the past week ... with friends	3.079	2.911	***	3.337	2.920	***	***	N.S.
During the past week ... with your family	2.678	3.421	***	2.999	3.559	***	***	***
Is there anybody you feel particularly close to	1.137	1.046	***	1.142	1.040	***	N.S.	N.S.
No. of informal helpers providing or currently	2.488	2.430	N.S.	2.125	2.889	***	***	***
No. of informal helpers relied on indefinitely	1.050	1.262	***	0.884	0.860	N.S.	***	***
When you have to make a decision	1.023	1.041	**	1.037	1.082	***	**	***

Table B8. Continued

	Baseline means			Follow-up means			Baseline to follow-up means	
	CCRC (N 1,570)	MA elders (N = 1,266)	Significance	CCRC (N 1,570)	MA elders (N = 1,266)	Significance	CCRC (N = 1,570)	MA elders (N = 1,266)
Unmet needs								
Would you say that you have [(1) Enough money to live on without any troubles . . . (4) Not enough to make ends meet]	1.163	1.676	***	1.173	1.692	***	N.S.	N.S.
No. of unmet needs reported by respondent [(0) None . . . (8) Eight]	0.136	0.069	***	0.218	0.129	***	***	***

Note. An asterisk (*) in the column indicates that the difference between the two groups is statistically different at the $p \leq 0.05$ probability level. Two asterisks (**) indicate statistical significance at the ≤ 0.01 level. Three asterisks (***) indicate statistical significance at the ≤ 0.001 level. N.S., not significant.

[a] (1) Self-sufficient in ADLs and IADLs (can have problem going out of house or being prevented from doing things would like to be doing). (2) Minimally sufficient: has one ADL or IADL problem and prevented from going out of house or doing things would like to be doing or has two ADL or IADL problems and not prevented from going out of house or doing things would like to be doing. (3) More severe: no ADL problem or one ADL problem and less than two IADL problems. (4) Most severe: more than one ADL problem or one ADL problem and more than one IADL problem.

[b] Items in ADL impairment index are: dressing, bathing, personal care, managing medications, transfer.

[c] Items in IADL impairment index are: doing ordinary housework, taking out garbage, and needs help most or all of the time with light housekeeping, chores, meal preparation, shopping and small errands, and transportation.

[d] Items in mobility impairment scale: uses walker/wheelchair, problem in climbing stairs, wheeling twenty feet; wheeling a half-mile, walking twenty feet, walking a half-mile (wheeling not considered a problem area if walks a half-mile).

[e] Does or does not know year, month, address.

[f] Number of helpers up to four.

References

American Association of Homes for the Aging. 1987. *Guidelines for Regulation of Continuing Care Retirement Communities*. Washington, D.C.: American Association of Homes for the Aging.

American Association of Homes for the Aging and Ernst and Whinney. 1987. *Continuing Care Retirement Communities: An Industry in Action*. Washington, D.C.: American Association of Homes for the Aging.

American Association of Homes for the Aging and Ernst and Young. 1992. *Continuing Care Retirement Communities: An Industry in Action*. Vol. 1, *Overview and Developing Trends*. Washington, D.C.: American Association of Homes for the Aging.

American Association of Homes and Services for the Aging. 1994. *Continuing Care Retirement Community Consumers Directory*. Washington, D.C.: American Association of Homes and Services for the Aging.

Anderson, G., and Knickman, J. R. 1984. Patterns of expenditures among high utilizers of medical care services. *Medical Care* 22:143–49.

Barbaro, E. L., and Noyes, L. E. 1984. A wellness program for a life care community. *Gerontologist* 24:568–71.

Bishop, C. E. 1988. Use of nursing care in continuing care retirement communities. In: Scheffler, R. M., and Rossiter, L. F. (eds.). *Advances in Health Economics and Health Services Research*. Greenwich, Conn.: JAF Press, 149–62.

Cassel, E. J. 1993. *The Consumers' Directory of Continuing Care Retirement Communities*. Washington, D.C.: American Association of Homes for the Aging.

Cohen, D. 1980. Continuing care communities for the elderly: Potential pitfalls and proposal regulations. *University of Pennsylvania Law Review* 128:883–936.

Cohen, M. A. 1988. Life care: New options for financing and delivering long-term care. *Health Care Financing Review* (suppl.) 10:139–44.

Cohen, M. A., Tell, E. J., Batten, H. L., and Larson, M. M. 1988a. Attitudes toward joining continuing care retirement communities. *Gerontologist* 28:637–43.

Cohen, M. A., Tell, E. J., Bishop, C. E., Wallack, S. S., and Branch, L. G. 1989. Patterns of nursing home use in a prepaid managed care system: The continuing care retirement community. *Gerontologist* 29:74-81.

Cohen, M. A., Tell, E. J., Greenberg, J. N., and Wallack, S. S. 1987. The financial capacity of the elderly to insure for long-term care. *Gerontologist* 27:494–502.

Cohen, M. A., Tell, E. J., and Wallack, S. 1988b. The risk factors of nursing home entry among residents of six continuing care retirement communities. *Journal of Gerontology Social Sciences* 43:S15–21.

Continuing Care Accreditation Commission. 1987. *Continuing Care Accreditation Handbook.* Washington, D.C.: American Association of Homes for the Aging.

Densen, P. M., Shapiro, S., and Einhorn, M. 1959. Concerning high and low utilizers of services in a medical plan, and the persistence of utilization levels over a three-year period. *Milbank Memorial Fund Quarterly* 37:217–50.

Elliott, F. E., and Elliott, S. H. 1985. Evolving management structure: A case study of a life care village at Pine Run, Doylestown, Bucks County, Pennsylvania. *Journal of Housing for the Elderly* 3:73–98.

Estes, C. L. 1993. The aging enterprise revisited. *Gerontologist* 33:292–98.

Falconer, J., Naughton, B. J., Hughes, S. L., Chang, R. W., Singer, R. H., and Sinacore, J. M. 1992. Self-reported functional status predicts change in level of care in independent living residents of a continuing care retirement community. *Journal of American Geriatrics Society* 40:255–58.

Feinauer, D. 1987. Movement of residents through multilevel lifetime care facilities: A Markovian matrix analysis. *Journal of Applied Gerontology* 6:313–31.

Fillenbaum, G. G. 1981. Portrait of a lifecare community: An alternate living arrangement for the elderly. *Center Reports on Advances in Research.* Durham, N.C.: Duke University Center for the Study of Aging and Human Development, 5(April):2.

German, P. S., and Fried, L. P. 1989. Prevention and the elderly: Public health issues and strategies. *Annual Review of Public Health* 10:319–32.

Gornick, M., Greenberg, J., Eggers, P., and Dobson, A. 1985. Twenty years of Medicare and Medicaid: Covered populations, use of benefits, and program expenditures. *Health Care Financing Review* (suppl.) 77:13-59.

Gunts, E. 1994. Housing the elderly. *Architecture* 83(October):82–87.

Hartwigsen, G. 1984–1985. The appeal of the life care facility to the older widow. *Journal of Housing* 2:63–75.

Helbing, C., Latta, V. B., and Keene, R. E. 1991. Medicare expenditures for physician and supplier services, 1970–88. *Health Care Financing Review* 12:109–20.

Higgens, D. P. 1992. Continuum of care retirement facilities: Perspectives on advance fee arrangements. *Journal of Housing for the Elderly* 10:77–92.

Hunt, M. E., Feldt, A. G., Marans, R. W., Pastalan, L. A., and Vakalo, K. L. 1983. Continuing care retirement communities: Friendship Village, Schaumberg, Illinois. *Journal of Housing for the Elderly* 1:205–47.

Hypertension Detection and Follow-up Program Cooperative Group. 1977. Blood pressure studies in fourteen communities: A two-stage screen for hypertension. *Journal of the American Medical Association* 237:2385–91.

Institute of Medicine. 1990. *The Second Fifty Years: Promoting Health and Preventing Disability.* Washington, D.C.: National Academy Press.

Kane, R. L., Kane, R. A., and Arnold, S. B. 1985. Prevention and the elderly: Risk factors. *Health Services Research* 19:945–1006.

Kaplan, G. A., and Haan, M. N. 1989. Is there a role for prevention among the elderly?: Epidemiological evidence from the Alameda County study. In: Ory, M. G., and Bonds, K. (eds.). *Aging and Health Care: Social Science Policy Perspectives.* New York: Routledge, 27–51.

Latta, V. B., and Keene, R. E. 1990. Use and cost of short-stay hospital inpatient services under Medicare, 1988. *Health Care Financing Review* 12:91–99.

Lavizzo-Mourey, R., and Diserens, D. 1992. Preventive care for the elderly. In: Somers, A. R., and Spears, N. L. (eds.). *The Continuing Care Retirement Community: A Significant Option for Long Term Care.* New York: Springer Publishing Co., 53–70.

Lawton, M. P. 1988. Three functions of the residential environment. *Journal of Housing for the Elderly* 5:35–50.

Leaverton, P. E., Havlik, R. J., and Ingster-Moore, L. M. 1990. Coronary heart disease and hypertension. In: Cornoni-Huntley, J. C., Huntley, R. R., and Feldman, J. J. (eds.). *Health Status and Well-being of the Elderly: National Health and Nutrition Examination Survey.* Vol. 1, *Epidemiologic Follow-up Study.* New York: Oxford University Press, 53–70.

Longino, C. F., Jr. 1986. *The Oldest Americans: State Profiles for Data Based Planning.* Coral Gables, Fla.: Center for Social Research in Aging, University of Miami.

Lubitz, J., and Prihoda, R. 1984. The use and costs of Medicare services in the last two years of life. *Health Care Financing Review* 5:117–31.

Lubitz, J. D., and Riley, G. F. 1993. Trends in Medicare payments in the last year of life. *New England Journal of Medicine* 328:1092–96.

Magan, G. G. 1993. New retirement communities offer equity, services and tax shelters. *Housing Reports.* Washington, D.C.: American Association of Retired Persons, 5–6.

Marans, R. W., Hunt, M. E., and Vakalo, K. L. 1984. Retirement communities. In: Altman, I., Lawton, M. P., and Wohlwill, J. F. (eds.). *Elderly People and the Environment.* New York: Plenum Press, 57–93.

McCall, N. 1984. Utilization and costs of Medicare services by beneficiaries in their last year of life. *Medical Care* 22:329–42.

McCall, N., and Wai, H. S. 1983. An analysis of the use of medical services by the continuously enrolled aged. *Medical Care* 21:567–85.

Morris, J. N., and Sherwood, S. 1975. A retesting and modification of the Philadelphia Geriatric Center Morale Scale. *Journal of Gerontology* 30:77–84.

Morrison, A. S., Brisson, J., and Khalid, N. 1988. Breast cancer incidence and mortality in the breast cancer detection demonstration project. *Journal of the National Cancer Institute* 80:1540–47.

Morrison, I. A., Bennett, R., Frisch, S., and Gurland, B. J. (eds). 1986. *Continuing Care Retirement Communities.* New York: Haworth Press.

Mossey, J. A., and Shapiro, E. 1985. Physician use by the elderly over an eight-year period. *American Journal of Public Health* 75:1333-34.

Muller, C., Mandelblatt, J., and Schechter, C. B. 1990. *Cost and Effectiveness of Cervical Cancer Screening in Elderly Women*. OTA-BP-H-65. Washington, D.C.: U.S. Government Printing Office.

Netting, F. E. 1991. Older women in continuing care retirement communities. *Journal of Women and Aging* 3:23-35.

Netting, F. E., and Wilson, C. C. 1994. CCRC oversight: Implications for public regulation and private accreditation. *Journal of Applied Gerontology* 13: 250-66.

Netting, F. E., Wilson, C. C., Stearns, L. R., and Branch, L. G. 1990. CCRC statutes: The oversight of long-term care service delivery. *Journal of Applied Gerontology* 9:139-56.

Netting, F. E., Wilson, C. C., Stearns, L. R., and Branch, L. G. 1992. State unit on aging involvement with continuing care retirement community legislation. *Journal of Applied Gerontology* 11:262-82.

Newcomer, R., and Preston, S. 1994. Relationships between acute care and nursing unit use in two continuing care retirement communities. *Research on Aging* 16:280-300.

Palmore, E. 1970. Health practices and illness among the aged. *Gerontologist* 10:313-16.

Pastalan, L. A. 1989. Introduction. *Journal of Housing for the Elderly* 5:1-3.

Rabins, P. V., Storer, D. J., and Lawrence, M. P. 1992. Psychiatric consultation to a continuing care retirement community. *Gerontologist* 32:126-28.

Ransohoff, D. F., and Lang, M. D. 1993. Sigmoidoscopic screening in the 1990s. *Journal of the American Medical Association* 269:1278-81.

Raper, A. T., and Kalicki, A. C. (eds.). 1988. American Association of Homes for the Aging. *National Continuing Care Directory*. Washington, D.C.: American Association of Retired Persons.

Riley, G., Lubitz, J., Prihoda, R., and Rabey, E. 1987. The use and costs of Medicare services by cause of death. *Inquiry* 24:233-44.

Ruchlin, H. S. 1987. A financial profile of continuing care retirement communities. *Healthcare Financial Management* 41:54-61.

Ruchlin, H. S. 1988. Continuing care retirement communities: An analysis of financial viability and health care coverage. *Gerontologist* 28:156-62.

Ruchlin, H. S., Morris, S., and Morris, J. N. 1993. Resident medical care utilization patterns in continuing care retirement communities. *Health Care Financing Review* 14:151-67.

Selby, J. V. 1993. How should we screen for colorectal cancer? *Journal of the American Medical Association* 269:1294-95.

Shapiro, S., Venet, W., Strax, P., Venet, L., and Roeser, R. 1985. Selection, follow-up, and analysis in the health insurance plan study: A randomized trial with breast cancer screening. In: Garfinkel, L., Ochs, O., and Mushinski, M. (eds.). *Selection, Follow-up, and Analysis in Prospective Studies: A Workshop*. National Cancer Institute Monograph 87. Washington, D.C.: U.S. Government Printing Office, 65-74.

SHEP Cooperative Research Group. 1991. Prevention of stroke by antihypertensive drug treatment in older persons with isolated systolic hypertension: Final results of the systolic hypertension in the elderly program. *Journal of the American Medical Association* 265:3255–64.

Sherwood, C. C., Sherwood, S., and Morris, S. A. 1993. CCRC residents and their age peers in the general population. Paper presented at the 46th Annual Scientific Meeting of the Gerontological Society of America, New Orleans, La.

Sherwood, S., Gutkin, C. E., Lewis, T. G., Sr., and Sherwood, C. C. 1988. Housing alternatives for an aging society. In: *Legislative Agenda for an Aging Society, 1988 and Beyond*. Proceedings of a Congressional Forum by the Select Committee on Aging, House of Representatives and the Special Committee on Aging, United States Senate, November 1987 (House Select Committee on Aging, Publication 100-664; Senate Special Committee on Aging Publication 100-J). Washington, D.C.: U.S. Government Printing Office.

Sherwood, S., and Morris, S. In press. Congregate housing. In: van Vliet, W. (ed.). *Encyclopedia of Housing.* New York: Garland Publishing, Inc.

Sherwood, S., Ruchlin, H. S., and Sherwood, C. C. 1989. CCRCs: An option for aging in place. In: Tilson, D. (ed.). *Aging in Place: Supporting the Frail Elderly in Residential Environments.* Glenview, Ill.: Scott, Foresman and Co., 125–64.

Silverman, H. A. 1991. Medicare-covered skilled nursing facility services, 1967–88. *Health Care Financing Review* 12:103–8.

Somers, A. R. 1993. Life care: A viable approach for long-term care for the elderly. *Journal of the American Geriatrics Society* 41:188–91.

Somers, A. R., and Livengood, W. S. 1992. Long-term care for the elderly: Major developments of the last ten years. *Pride Institute Journal of Long Term Home Health Care* 2:6–18.

Somers, A. R., and Spears, N. L. 1992. *The Continuing Care Retirement Community: A Significant Option for Long Term Care.* New York: Springer Publishing Co.

Stacey-Konnert, C., and Pynoos, J. 1992. Friendship and social networks in a continuing care retirement community. *Journal of Applied Gerontology* 11:298–313.

Stenback, A., Kumpulaines, M., and Van Konen, M. L. 1978. Illness and health behavior in septuagenarians. *Journal of Gerontology* 33:57–61.

Stephens, M. A. P., Kinney, J. M., and McNeer, A. E. 1986. Accommodative housing: Social integration of residents with physical limitations. *Gerontologist* 26:176–79.

Tell, E. J., and Cohen, M. A. 1990. Continuing care retirement communities. *Generations* 14:55–59.

Thompson, B., and Swisher, M. 1983. An assessment, using the Multiphasic Environmental Assessment Procedure (MEAP) of a rural life care residential center for the elderly. *Journal of Housing for the Elderly* 1:41–56.

Topolnicki, D. M. 1985. The broken promise of life care communities. *Money* 14:150–57.

U.S. Congress, Office of Technology Assessment. 1985. *Technology and Aging in America*. OTA-BA-264. Washington, D.C.: U.S. Government Printing Office.

U.S. Department of Health and Human Services. 1987. Health statistics on older persons, 1986: Analytical and epidemiological studies. Series 3, no. 5. In: *Vital and Health Statistics*. DHHS Publication (PHS) 87-1409. Washington, D.C.: U.S. Government Printing Office.

U.S. Department of Health and Human Services. 1991. *Healthy People 200: National Health Promotion and Disease Prevention Objectives*. DHHS Publication (PHS) 91-50213. Washington, D.C.: U.S. Government Printing Office.

U.S. Department of Health and Human Services, Social Security Administration, Office of Policy, Office of Research, Statistics, and International Policy. 1985. SSA Publication 13-11871. *Income of the Population 55 and Over, 1984*. Washington, D.C.: U.S. Government Printing Office.

U.S. Senate, Special Committee on Aging. 1983. *Life Care Communities: Promises and Problems*. 98th Congress. Washington, D.C.: U.S. Government Printing Office.

U.S. Senate, Special Committee on Aging. 1988. *Developments in Aging, 1987*. Volume 1. 100th Congress, Second Session. Washington, D.C.: U.S. Government Printing Office, 183.

Veterans Administration Cooperative Study Group on Antihypertensive Agents. 1970. Effects of treatment on morbidity in hypertension: Results in patients with diastolic blood pressure averaging 90 through 114 mmHg. *Journal of the American Medical Association* 213:1143–52.

Weeden, J. P., Newcomer, R. J., and Byerts, T. O. 1986. Housing and shelter for frail and nonfrail elders: Current options and future directions. In: Newcomer, R. J., Lawton, M. P., and Byerts, T. O. (eds.). *Housing an Aging Society*. New York: Van Nostrand Reinhold Company.

White, L. R., Losonczy, K. G., and Wolf, P. A. 1990. Cerebrovascular disease. In: Cornoni-Huntley, J. C., Huntley, R. R., and Feldman, J. J. (eds.). *Health Status and Well-being of the Elderly: National Health and Nutrition Examination Survey*. Vol. 1, *Epidemiologic Follow-up Study*. New York: Oxford University Press, 115–35.

Wingard, D. L., Berkman, L. F., and Branf, R. J. 1982. A multivariate analysis of health-related practices: A nine-year follow-up of the Alameda County study. *American Journal of Epidemiology* 116:765–75.

Winklevoss, H. E., Powell, A. V., Cohen, D. C., and Trueblood-Raper, A. 1984. *Continuing Care Retirement Communities: An Empirical, Financial, and Legal Analysis*. Homewood, Ill.: Richard D. Irwin, Inc., 23.

Index

ABOUT THE AUTHORS

Sylvia Sherwood, Ph.D., is Director of Housing and Long-term Care Research, Research and Training Institute, Hebrew Rehabilitation Center for Aged, Boston, Massachusetts; and Clinical Professor, Community Health, Brown University Medical School, Providence, Rhode Island.

Hirsch S. Ruchlin, Ph.D., is Professor of Economics in Public Health and Medicine, Cornell University Medical College, New York, New York.

Clarence C. Sherwood, Ph.D., is Professor Emeritus, Boston University School of Social Work, and Consultant, Research and Training Institute, Hebrew Rehabilitation Center for Aged, Boston, Massachusetts.

Shirley A. Morris, M.A., is Research Associate, Research and Training Institute, Hebrew Rehabilitation Center for Aged, Boston, Massachusetts.